APHASIA THERAPEUTICS

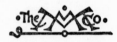

THE MACMILLAN COMPANY
NEW YORK · CHICAGO
DALLAS · ATLANTA · SAN FRANCISCO

**THE MACMILLAN COMPANY
OF CANADA, LIMITED**
TORONTO

MARY COATES LONGERICH, Ph.D.

JEAN BORDEAUX, Ph.D.

APHASIA

THERAPEUTICS

FOREWORDS BY
HAROLD ROSEN, PH.D., M.D.
AND FRED B. MOOR, M.D.

THE MACMILLAN COMPANY - NEW YORK

1954

FOREWORD

APHASIA, BY DEFINITION, IMPLIES INJURY TO NERVE CELLS
and association fibers. Head injuries, to mention one cause
only, are all too common in these days of high-powered driv-
ing and even higher-powered cold warfare. And actual organic deficit cannot be made up: brain cells, as is well
known, do not regenerate.

But aphasia involves more than merely loss of speech
through destruction of cells in one part or other of either hemisphere. Psychiatrists are not infrequently asked to see patients whose personality problems make effective aphasia
therapeutics impossible unless treatment of their emotional
difficulties be initiated. In addition, the reaction of the patient to his inability to communicate adequately with friends
and family is often of prime importance. This must, in fact,
almost inevitably be taken into consideration if the patient
is to be helped to function on as high a level as possible in
view of the cerebral damage actually sustained and not or-
ganically compensated. Retraining of the aphasic patient in
the ways of speech may therefore be a long-continuing, exceedingly complex process requiring special ability, spe-
cialized knowledge, and especial patience on the part of his
therapist. And unfortunately there are all too few who
are competently trained in the complex field of aphasia
therapeutics.

The literature on the subject is vast. The War of 1812, for
instance, was barely over when Gall first described speech

v

loss with right hemiplegia, and the Civil War was just drawing to a close when Armand Trousseau introduced the term
aphasia to medical and psychological science. Concepts have
long since been critically studied and investigated; yet theoretical explanations even today are not too clear. Aphasic
phenomena are still poorly understood. This is despite the
mass of detail which, to the student of the subject, occasionally seems almost overwhelming.

Drs. Longerich and Bordeaux have accomplished an almost Herculean task in organizing in this book, clearly and
readably and almost in outline form, those aspects of the
subject which are of clinical importance in the field of aphasia therapeutics. Theoretical material is summarized, but
only insofar as it helps make understandable—and possible
—treatment of the aphasic phenomena themselves, once the
patient has weathered the acute medical or surgical condition responsible for his speech and linguistic difficulties. Further, they stress the need for considering each patient not as
a symptom complex but as a person in his own right. By im-
plication, the need for responsible care—and caution—is emphasized. This book, therefore, becomes of prime importance
to the specialist in aphasia therapeutics. It is, in addition, of
much more than mere general interest to the family physician, the neurologist, the psychologist, and the psychiatrist.
For all in intimate daily contact with the overlapping fields
of organic and psychosomatic medicine, the implications of
this work, with its emphasis on the need for emotional re-
education along with medical treatment in the handling of
the aphasic patient, cannot be overemphasized. And for
those of us who are concerned primarily with the problems
posed in the study of the various forms of verbal communication between one person and another, this book will prove of
prime interest with its clear organization and its emphasis on
what can be done—and how—to help the aphasic patient

again enter into meaningful communication with his fellow human beings.

It has been a privilege and a pleasure to read the manuscript of this book. It is an honor to be permitted to write this foreword.

HAROLD ROSEN, PH.D., M.D.
Henry Phipps Psychiatric Clinic
The Johns Hopkins Hospital
Baltimore 5, Maryland

FOREWORD

THE RESTORATION OF THE PATIENT, HANDICAPPED BY DISEASE or injury, to the best physical and mental state which it is possible for him to attain, is known as medical rehabilitation. In the rehabilitation of patients with brain damage, aphasia therapy often plays an important role. There are few things more frustrating to a handicapped individual than his inability to express himself in understandable speech or to comprehend the import of the speech of others. On the other hand, there is nothing which improves the mental outlook of these patients so profoundly as the process of total rehabilitation including speech therapy.

In the United States during the past half century, modern preventive and curative medicine have added 20 years to the average span of human life. Many of the infectious diseases have been conquered, but this is not an unmixed blessing. We are left with an aging population in which the chronic degenerative diseases predominate. Among these, atherosclerosis with its coronary occlusions, cerebral thromboses, and cerebral hemorrhages rank high as a cause of death or disability. Many of these patients have aphasia caused by damage to the association area of the brain. In these often neglected individuals, the earlier rehabilitation procedures are initiated, the better is the outlook for restoration.

In the cerebral palsies of childhood, a variety of speech difficulties are encountered. Approximately 60 per cent of these children are either mentally normal or are not impaired sufficiently to interfere with educational procedures. The recent emphasis on the rehabilitation of cerebral palsied children places a further responsibility upon our all too few speech pathologists.

Trauma to the brain, whether it be unavoidably produced during the surgical removal of a brain tumor or by one of the accidents so common in our industrialized civilization, may cause impairment or loss of the function of speech. Speech therapy by a competent speech pathologist is often essential for maximum recovery.

The authors of *Aphasia Therapeutics* have produced a volume which should be exceedingly useful to the graduate student of medicine, especially in the fields of neurology and physical medicine, as well as to the student of speech pathology. It is remarkable for the absence of vague generalizations which leave the student with hazy concepts of actual techniques.

The text is concise yet replete with detailed instruction as to just how speech rehabilitation is done. The importance of careful preliminary diagnostic study as a basis for aphasia therapeutics has been commendably stressed. The book is a valuable addition to the literature on aphasia therapy as well as to the broader field of rehabilitation.

FRED B. MOOR, M.D.
Professor of Therapeutics, School of Medicine
and Director of School of Physical Therapy
College of Medical Evangelists, Los Angeles

PREFACE

DURING PANEL DISCUSSIONS AT SENIOR MEDICAL CONFERENCES directed by Dr. Fred B. Moor at the School of Medicine of the College of Medical Evangelists, Los Angeles, Dr. Cyril B. Courville repeatedly emphasized to the graduating students in medicine (and to the visiting lecturers in orthopaedics, physiatrics, and logopaedics) the vital necessity for a most careful diagnosis and adequate treatment which were essential in the correct handling of aphasia cases. One of the authors of this book (M. C. L.) was a member of those panels and from time to time discussed with the panel lecturers the need for further research and information in this field of aphasia therapeutics. From these discussions the idea for this book germinated.

The other author (J. B.) has served as visiting lecturer in speech to the General Practice Section of the Los Angeles County Medical Association, and at various sessions discussed with physicians in attendance the need for clinical research in aphasia therapy. Some of our outstanding neurologists, neurosurgeons, psychiatrists, and physiatrists are so busy with hospital and staff work that they cannot find time to devote to clinical research with aphasics. They expressed the wish that psychologists would make such studies under supervision of the staff of the aphasia sections in hospitals.

The encouragement of such men as Dr. Fred B. Moor and Dr. Charles Le Roy Lowman stimulated the authors to report their findings in this text, *Aphasia Therapeutics*.

ACKNOWLEDGMENTS

The authors are deeply grateful to Dr. J. M. Nielsen, Dr. Cullen Ward Irish, Dr. Harold Rosen, Dr. Fred B. Moor, Dr. Robert C. Robb, Dr. William G. Hardy, and Dr. Sol Charen for their reading of the manuscript and for the helpful suggestions they have made. We also wish to express our appreciation to Carol Angel, R.N., and Joyce Regal for their assistance in compiling data for the therapy section; to Helen Frantz and Carol Blaney who helped to arrange the index; and to our secretaries, Elizabeth Hadley and Elizabeth Hurt, for the typing of the manuscript.

M. C. L.
J. B.

CONTENTS

APHASIA THERAPEUTICS

CHAPTER I

INTRODUCTION

PRIOR TO THE TWENTIETH CENTURY, THERAPEUTIC RETRAIN-
ing techniques used with aphasic patients resembled those
used in training young children. Emphasis was placed almost
entirely upon the use of the five senses and this methodology
tended to be artificial. Consequently, little progress was made
in aphasia therapeutics and various workers in the field
looked upon the retraining of the aphasic—particularly the
apoplectic—as rather hopeless.

Mills's paper[1] in 1904 threw new light upon the treatment
of the aphasic. His study pointed out that the aphasic's earlier
life experience (along with his already organized brain functioning and particular speech loss) presented a more intricate
problem than that of teaching a child. In addition, he felt that
the limitation of the aphasic's training to Pavlovian methodologies alone usually proved inadequate. We believe
Mills's work marked one of the turning points in aphasia
therapy. (See page 109.)

The large number of traumatic aphasic cases produced by
World War I led medical people to realize the need for more
satisfactory training devices. As a result, several important
contributions were made in the field of aphasia therapy,
chiefly that by Kurt Goldstein, *Die Behandlung, Fürsorge und
Begutachtung der Hirnverletzten.*[2] Goldstein asserted that the

[1] Mills, Charles: "Treatment of Aphasia by Training," *J.A.M.A.*, **43**:1940–49,
1904.
[2] Goldstein, Kurt: *Die Behandlung, Fürsorge und Begutachtung der Hirnverletzten.* F. C. W. Vogel, Leipzig, 1919.

1

first requisite in aphasia therapy is a thorough examination (see Chapter V, "Appraisal of the Patient's Capacities"); furthermore, that it was essential to determine first of all the limits of the patient's abilities in the various performances, the nature of his difficulties, and then outline the therapeutic procedures most apt to alleviate the aphasic problems. Goldstein believed the aphasic's rehabilitation consists in relearning specific responses (providing it is indicated in the particular case) and in learning compensatory techniques for those lost or disturbed.[3]

Goldstein's more recent contributions, *Aftereffects of Brain Injuries in War* and *Language and Language Disturbances*, together with Weisenburg and McBride's *Aphasia*, Granich's *Aphasia*, and Wepman's *Recovery from Aphasia*, have put even greater emphasis upon aphasia therapy. These were not only distinct contributions to the literature but stimulated further research in this field.

The U.S. Veterans Administration recently published statistics revealing that some 400,000 aphasia cases exist at the present time in the United States alone, and that number is increasing alarmingly. A vast amount of research has been done in the past on the organic aspects of aphasia, but little has been done on the functional aspects. Trained and well-experienced speech pathologists and clinical psychologists are needed who can and will work closely with the medical profession to reinvestigate functional aphasia.

[3] *Ibid.*

CHAPTER II

EARLY IDEAS ON APHASIA

SINCE IT IS ALMOST IMPOSSIBLE TO PUT A DETAILED HISTORY drawn from all available literature on aphasia into one volume, we have elected to review briefly earlier contributions and the major viewpoints therein regarding speech and language problems and therapy. We have tried to cover all worth-while contributions of neurologists, psychiatrists, speech pathologists, and clinical psychologists.

Prior to the early 1800's, there was little or no attempt to localize speech problems in specific cerebral areas. Flourens believed the entire brain served one and the same function and declared any part of it could take over the functioning in lieu of any other part where there was injury or disease to the brain cells. Gall of Vienna attempted to localize the speech faculty by placing it in the area of the brain just above the eyes, and this theory was accepted by Spurzheim. The two became so fanatic about the idea that they wound up as out-and-out phrenologists.

A French physician by the name of Marc Dax noticed that among patients who suffered a language loss, there was usually also, more or less, hemiplegia on the right side of the body but seldom on the left. The Parisian doctor Bouillaud decided the faculty of language must lie in the frontal lobes of the brain, but all these mentioned theories were attacked by Lordat who had become aphasic and then wrote a book on the subject. He described how he "knew" words but could not use them properly, nor could he understand others. While aphasic, Lordat was unable to read his own writing. His description indicates he probably experienced receptive (sensory) aphasia due (so he asserted) to asynergy of the speech muscles.

Dax again came out with some ideas on aphasia and put the speech faculty in the left side of the brain. He made this assertion after some 30 years of observing aphasic problems. Bouillaud still maintained his theory in opposition to Dax, so Cruveilhier and Broca tried to settle the arguments by an autopsy which apparently showed Bouillaud was right. Broca then attempted to localize speech at the base of the third left frontal convolution and was of the opinion that a right-handed individual with an injury to the third left convolution would have a disturbance in language. Those patients having a lesion in the right hemisphere would not. He termed such loss of function "aphémie." Associated with Broca was Trousseau, who would not accept Broca's localization theory. As a result, two schools of thought—structural and dynamic—arose and are in existence today.

Trousseau learned during his researches that "aphémie" meant "infamy" while "aphasia" meant "speechlessness," being so used before the days of Christ. Broca accepted this finding and "aphasia" is the term generally used today.

In the mid-1800's Wyllie expressed his idea that the speech faculty is both supramotor and suprasensory. This was the first attempt to set up an anatomical-physiological concept of aphasia. Moxon, Liepmann, Hughlings Jackson, Ogle, Wernicke, Kussmaul, Munk, Hitzig, Luciani, Seppilli, all inclined to the anatomical viewpoint. Charcot and Freud felt that aphasia might be psychic, although both were willing to accept the localization theories previously advanced.

Dejerine, Starr, Maudsley, Marie, all opposed localization hypotheses, yet they and their followers believed language disturbances were more or less matters of physiology and anatomy. Hughlings Jackson believed firmly in a psychological explanation. His attitude was bolstered by Head, Pick, Goldstein, Weisenburg, and McBride. The last three decades have brought various changes in viewpoints, as well as confirmation of some old ideas on aphasia. Henschen and Head wasted much time in opposition to each other. Finally Head began a completely new study on patients, building up enormous amounts of substantiating data to prove that his anatomical-physiological viewpoint was the only correct one. He furnished some helpful semantic ideas for use in treating the aphasic, but the Germans were able to show his physiological stand lacked merit.

In opposition to Head, the studies of Henschen were based solely on autopsies. He discarded all psychological ideas. His monograph ran to three volumes and covered over 1500 cases, as well as a survey of all the literature of the world on aphasia. The monograph was extremely bulky and was published in four languages. Even neurologists hesitated to delve into its contents.

The eminent neurologist J. M. Nielsen believed Henschen had made a real contribution. The more Nielsen studied and compared the written data with observations in his daily practice, the more he felt a small and modern monograph should be brought out. His outstanding book, *Agnosia, Apraxia, Aphasia*, was first issued in 1936 and a second edition came out in 1946. Such men as Dr. Rupert B. Raney, Dr. Mandel Cohen, Dr. Stanley Cobb, all endorsed Nielsen's viewpoint. He was primarily interested in cerebral localization in neurological diagnosis. The result was a volume of major importance to all therapists handling aphasia cases.

The atomistic psychologists presently feel that at least certain types of aphasia have to do with the dissociation of object images and word images, and that particular language is disturbed or damaged when there is an injury to a particular area of the brain. In the larger percentage of aphasia cases, brain disturbances occur in the dominant hemisphere—usually the left, hence brain damage is most likely to be found on the opposite side to handedness. Only in a very small percentage of aphasia cases does handedness fail to correspond with the speech localization.

All problems involving aphasia seem to have psychic, as well as anatomical involvements. Not only does the patient suffer from a localized defect, but he has trouble in assuming voluntary attitudes and extreme difficulty in coming to terms with his environment. (See pages 9–60.) The entire psychic personality is involved, as well as his physical self. Readers interested in prior theories may find the Bibliography (pages 169–74) helpful.

CHAPTER III

APHASIA TERMINOLOGY

THE AUTHORS DEFINE "APHASIA" AS A DISTURBANCE IN ABIL-
ity to recognize audible and visible communicative symbols,
or to produce mental concepts in well-planned words, phrases,
sentences, or paragraphs by means of speech or writing.
Aphasia is a basic disruption of the individual's organization
of speech and language demonstrating almost any combination of numerous aphasic symptoms. By the term "speech"
we refer to the voice and to the bodily actions an individual
uses to influence the behavior of others. The term "language"
comprises the words, phrases, and sentences expressed by
means of speech or writing. The disturbance is not due solely
to a defect of the peripheral sense organs or to impaired innervation of the speech musculature. The term "aphasia" is
used here in its broadest sense to include all aspects of the
problem.

There are two levels of aphasia observable in most cases.
The higher level pertains to that aspect where language is
limited in amount or degree rather than in quality. On this
upper aphasic level the patient may be totally unable to express himself through oral speech or in writing. The lower
level concerns those aspects of aphasia in which motor and
sensory symptoms are so marked as to be easily discernible.

Primarily, aphasia is a problem in association. Most aphasics are disturbed both in understanding and in expressing
mental concepts. However, one difficulty may seem more severe than the other. The aphasic state usually will appear

7

either as more *receptive* or more *expressive*, i.e., primarily sensory or motor in character depending upon the location of the lesion. The use of language is a complex process and its disorders involve more than the loss of one specific function. Aphasia, therefore, usually implicates a combination of activities. Rarely does an aphasia appear in isolated form since nearly all types overlap.

Aphasia must also be considered in correlation with the agnosia and apraxia aspects of the problem. By agnosia we refer to disturbances in recognizing words or objects; by apraxia we mean impairment in the ability to carry out a motor act even though there may be no paresis of the musculature. Aphasia is agnosic when due to receptive difficulties and apraxic if caused by expressive disturbances. (See pages 9–60.)

Nearly every aphasic suffers more or less amnesic loss and has difficulty in associating an object with the appropriate word or symbol. Finding a word to express his mental concept of the object becomes a problem, and this aspect sometimes is the most noticeable symptom. However, the pure form of amnesic aphasia is rare, although it appears to some degree in the majority of expressive and receptive aphasics. Amnesic aphasia (however slight) is a problem common to practically all aphasics, so we feel it should be considered as a separate major syndrome.

Aphasia herein has been approached from three major aspects: *receptive aphasia*, *expressive aphasia*, and *amnesic aphasia*. However, a study of aphasia symptomatology only from these three angles is not the sole concern of the aphasia therapist. Every aspect of the patient's behavior and all their interrelationships must be studied if the therapist is to help him.

CHAPTER IV

SYMPTOMATOLOGY

A. Etiological Background

DURING THE LATTER PART OF THE NINETEENTH CENTURY interest arose in the classical atomistic viewpoint of aphasia, according to which those disturbances were considered to be defects resulting from some form of lesion in the association fibers of the cortex which, in turn, gave rise to dissociations between the ideas of words and their corresponding object images as visualized or perceived by the aphasic.

But lesions in the association fibers must be differentiated from lesions in motor or sensory fibers because the latter are not known to produce aphasia. Where motor nerves have been damaged, the patient may be disturbed in motion and have difficulty in the use of his extremities or speech musculature. For example, he has difficulty in writing, running, walking, speaking, etc. When sensory nerves have been severed or damaged, the individual loses awareness of sensation, which is usually manifested by more or less deficiency in seeing, hearing, and the like.

Brain damage which creates mental deficiency or impaired innervation with paralysis of the writing or speech musculature (e.g., dysarthria) cannot be considered as aphasia. According to authorities, aphasia occurs where there is a damage to association nerve fibers pertaining to the functions of speech and language.

Most medical authorities believe damage occurs primarily from changes in the brain cells after their oxygen supply has been depleted. This is brought about in various ways. For example, any clot of blood or tumorous growth immediately creates pressure which might reduce the amount of blood entering the specific brain area. Other causes are: encephalitis, which creates an inflammation in the brain tissues and usually produces personality changes; epilepsy, which may likewise reduce oxygen in the brain.

Brain injuries may result from a ruptured blood vessel, caused by a blow on the head or during delivery. Brain hemorrhages cause deterioration in the affected area. Meningitis may also disturb the oxygen supply. Thrombosis is sometimes given as a cause. Little knowledge is available concerning the effects of even mild trauma to the mother's pelvic area. Certainly still less is known concerning intrauterine injections and other types of involvements (unknown actual illnesses of fetus) which also affect the brain.

Tertiary syphilis may attack the cerebral cortex. Paresis (parenchymatous syphilis of the brain) may develop unless adequate treatment is properly given. Along with such diseases as syphilis, the therapist ought to be informed about multiple sclerosis, which causes diffuse tissue degeneration that may involve the cerebrum, the spinal cord, and usually the brain stem. The end result is frequently more or less paralysis.

Traumas may cause some aphasia, as well as aphonia. Hysterical deafness or mutism may follow even a minor trauma in an emotionally unstable individual. Aphasias resulting from trauma vary so greatly among individuals that we purposely omit attempting to describe specific symptoms. Likewise, states of deliria may be accompanied by aphasic conditions which may be transient.

The general condition of the brain is highly important in all diagnosis. It is never amiss for the therapist to insist that a referred patient be checked with the electroencephalograph. Aphasia often shows up in epileptics, neurotics, alcoholics, psychotics, and those who have had some cerebrovascular accident. These conditions may be indicated by dysrhythmia revealed in an electroencephalogram.

The atomistic viewpoint considers the type of disturbance as presumably determined by the location of the brain lesion. It assumes that perception takes place only in the posterior central convolution while control of movement occurs in the anterior central convolution and speech in the left third convolution. This early concept is partially accepted by workers in the aphasic field today.[1]

It is generally believed that sensory loss is produced by a lesion of the posterior central convolution while disturbances of movement result from a lesion of the anterior central convolution, with language difficulties arising from a lesion of a particular part of the left third convolution. Jackson described such language disturbances (which are the direct result of impairment of the substratum) as *negative symptoms*.

Negative symptoms appear in certain aspects of initial motor aphasia in which the speech and/or language mechanisms lose only part of their functions. Recovery of these damaged functions may be brought about spontaneously by two factors:[2] first, by restriction of the damaged substratum; and secondly, through retraining brought about by demands from the environment. While recovery may occur during the first few weeks or months after injury, it may not occur for several months.

Spontaneous improvement is observed most often after surgery, although it sometimes follows drainage of abscesses and removal of bone splinters.[3] In other instances of expressive (motor) aphasia, the negative symptoms may be alleviated by systematic employment of speech exercises.

[1] Goldstein, Kurt: *Language and Language Disturbances*. Grune & Stratton, Inc., New York, 1948, p. 3.
[2] Goldstein, Kurt: *Aftereffects of Brain Injuries in War*. Grune & Stratton, Inc., New York, 1942, pp. 147–48.
[3] *Ibid.*, pp. 147–48.

(Goldstein[4] feels such therapeutics may resemble that of training a child.) Our observations indicate that aphasia therapy should not be limited only to such methods as those used in teaching the young child. Frequently other methods prove even more effective. (See the discussion of therapy under Expressive Aphasia, pages 135–54.) However, in certain cases of expressive aphasia, i.e., central motor aphasia, symptoms may not be eliminated or even mitigated by retraining of the damaged speech and language performances.

Wernicke was a strong adherent of the atomistic viewpoint but felt that aphasic symptoms could not always be explained from a localization viewpoint. He believed there were various factors (other than lesion) responsible for many aphasic difficulties.[5] Jackson similarly believed that aphasic disturbances could not be considered solely dependent on the location of the lesion in the cortex; that symptoms were not caused merely by impairment of structure. In fact, he was of the opinion that a lesion rarely manifested itself simply by a loss of performance. He felt that aphasic symptoms might result from an unimpaired area of the brain being isolated from an impaired one and asserted that each area (within the central nervous system) works in relation to the whole; hence abilities in one area must be influenced by function in other areas. If there was a loss of ability in one area, other dependent performances would be impeded as affected. Such symptoms were described by Jackson as *"positive" symptoms*, but Goldstein termed them "indirect" symptoms or "depending" symptoms, so called because they occurred as the result of dependence of an undamaged area on a damaged area—that is, resulting from an "irritation of the immediate neighborhood" or as a manifestation of Pavlov's Law of Peripheral Inhibition. Goldstein felt that symptoms resulting from

[4] *Ibid.*, pp. 147–48.
[5] Wernicke, C.: "The Symptom-Complex of Aphasia," in Church, Archibald (ed.): *Modern Clinical Medicine: Diseases of the Nervous System.* D. Appleton & Co., New York, 1907, pp. 265–324.

damage to the substratum by a scar or tumor often were relieved or improved after operation.[6] He further observed that symptoms actually might result from the aphasic's endeavor to prevent catastrophic reactions.

Goldstein pointed out that just because an aphasic does not carry out a certain piece of work or exercise is no reason to assume that he will always be unable to do it. Lack of ability to perform the task at that moment may be due to fear of being unable to do it—feeling that a mistake might throw him into a catastrophic situation. As a result, the patient builds up defensive performances to avoid such catastrophic reactions and the need of coming to terms with his environment. In Chapter V, "Appraisal of the Patient's Capacities," we point out that such apprehension of ability to perform a task may cause a patient to err; whereas, if the task is performed in a more relaxed environment, he would accomplish it. Such factors must be carefully considered when appraising the aphasic's abilities.

Thus it can be seen that behavioral deviations in brain damage cases may be brought about in entirely different ways. Summarizing, symptoms may be delineated according to cause, as follows:

1. Positive symptoms: those due to isolation of an unimpaired area from another impaired one.

2. Negative symptoms: those which are the specific result of impairment of the substratum. (Behavioral deviations resulting from the brain injury.)

3. Depending symptoms: those brought about as the result of the effect of a damaged area on an undamaged area.

[6] Goldstein, Kurt: *Language and Language Disturbances*. Grune & Stratton, Inc., New York, 1948, p. 9.

4. Fatigue symptoms: those which arise as a result of the patient's endeavor to prevent catastrophic reactions.

B. Psychological Symptomatology

From time to time in the journals and periodicals, articles have recently appeared in which were discussed so-called personality deviations displayed by brain-injured patients. These problems involving deterioration of attention, memory, and association of ideas commonly found in aphasic patients were mentioned by Pierre Marie[7] in 1906. Jackson[8] commented at length on the loss of higher intellectual controls and retrograde behavior he had observed in aphasics, expressing the belief that most aphasics retrogressed in personality and displayed primitive behavior resembling in many respects the development stages observable in young children.

Personality changes mainly considered in a casual observation to be due to aphasia, particularly in the presence of brain injury, may include numerous other symptoms of cerebral damage which may be due to pathological involvement. The aftereffects of strokelets often are exhibited by personality unconformities, seeming mental impairment, mental disturbances outside the speech and language area, and even physical disabilities. Superficially, the patient has aphasia, but it is essential to estimate his total defects in communicating with his environment, as well as his physical, emotional, and mental losses.

Relatives of aphasics frequently are concerned about such manifestations and may remark: "He's not the same as he used to be. He gets so annoyed when he can't use his right arm or leg [see page 4] and he doesn't seem to want to

[7] Marie, Pierre: "Revision de la question de l'aphasie," *Semaine méd.*, 1906.
[8] Head, Henry: "Hughlings Jackson on Aphasia and Kindred Disorders of Speech," *Brain*, 38:1–96, 1915.

help himself. We have to take care of him just like a baby. He's so cross and irritable now and doesn't seem to have the slightest interest in himself or in us. Once in a while he's co-operative but usually he's grouchy and inconsiderate. He gets sort of ugly and surly and cries a lot, and seems so discouraged. So are we!"

This picture of the aphasic is not unusual. Presumably an aphasic patient protected by his home environment ought to maintain consistency of behavior, but such is not the case. Many aphasic patients cooperate with the family at times and yet these same patients are easily upset, annoyed, or often display catastrophic reactions. Most investigators seem to agree as to the general nature of these. According to Goldstein, the patient "looks dazed, changes color, becomes agitated, anxious, begins to fumble, his pulse becomes irregular; a moment before amiable, he is now sullen, evasive, exhibits temper, and becomes aggressive."[9]

The Rorschach test was used by Z. A. Piotrowsky to study the behavior characteristics of aphasics. He pointed out that the individual tended to exhibit emotional instability, feelings of inadequacy, an inclination toward automatic verbalization, and lack of conformity in thought and behavior.[10] Similar findings were observed in World War II soldiers, as set forth in the 1945 U.S. Army report[11] which noted that brain-injured men generally revealed some or all of the following characteristics:

1. Reduced capacity for abstract thinking.
2. Disturbances of concentration and attention.

[9] Goldstein, Kurt: *Aftereffects of Brain Injuries in War.* Grune & Stratton, Inc., New York, 1942, p. 71.

[10] Piotrowsky, Z. A.: "Rorschach Method and Its Application in Organic Disturbances of the Central Nervous System," *Rorschach Res. Exch.*, 1:23, 1936–1937.

[11] Privileged U.S. Army Med. Dept. Comm.: "Aphasic Language Disorders," (October, 1945). Cited by J. M. Wepman in *Recovery from Aphasia.* The Ronald Press Co., New York, 1951, p. 26.

3. Memory defects.
4. Increased irritability, anxiety, euphoria, and various psychosomatic disturbances.
5. Reduced ability to adjust to new or strange situations.
6. Social withdrawal, shyness, and seclusiveness.
7. Strong tendency toward perseveration.

Brain damage definitely causes a delay in response to stimuli. When and if the response comes, the patient tends to perseverate. The aphasic manifests this by repeating a newly learned word over and over. George, a surgeon patient, was so delighted to learn to say *Carl* (the name of his physician associate), that he would say *Carl* over and over, and evidenced genuine pleasure while iterating. He exhibited a similar perseveration reaction after relearning the name *Si*—a nickname for another doctor friend.

Goldstein emphasized that aphasics experience a change in total personality following a traumatic onset. He was emphatic in affirming that the patient became a "changed person," but our clinical experience does not lead to that conclusion. We find most aphasics do *not* experience a change in basic personality following cerebral insult. Outward appearances may make the patient seem to be a "different person," but actually he is making characteristic adjustments to new physiological and psychological problems in accordance with present environmental stresses and in the light of his premorbid personality pattern. For example, the aphasic who formerly was a pessimistic or gloomy individual and "chronic" worrier, continually depressed by social contacts, is likely to respond similarly to his aphasic difficulty. On the other hand, the formerly optimistic person who took life in stride will react to a cerebral insult in a more objective manner. Thus, when George was asked by a group of physician friends when he was going to be able to talk, he "accidentally" came forth with the phrase "Some day." These are the patients who are inclined to accept more readily the fact that they have a serious problem. Such a person tries to face the problem squarely and sets out to do something about it. As pointed out in Chapter VI, "Speech and Language Prognosis," the willingness to attack the problem and improve himself stands the aphasic in excellent stead as he seeks to work through his difficulties.

An aphasic's personality is largely determined by his pre-morbid personality pattern and by the way he looks upon himself in the light of his present difficulties. Of course we omit here purposely organic factors such as arteriosclerosis, senile changes, and general mental deterioration. In the therapist's clinical picture the vital question is: "How does this particular aphasic appraise himself?" Rarely is an aphasic fully aware of the severity of his difficulty, a factor particularly noticeable in the case of a certain skilled surgeon who, at the beginning of his illness, did not even realize that the problem was an association loss. Prior to insult and the attendant illness, he would have readily discerned such a difficulty in any of his own patients. Aware only of feeling tremendously handicapped, he was completely scotomized to his own aphasia.

Ordinarily an aphasic recognizes that he has a problem and feels the need of adjusting to changed situations because life somehow is different. Because he does find life different, the therapist must discover what the aphasic regards as his greatest loss. In what area does this aphasic believe he needs the most help? Does he sense a greater loss in the area of speech? language? writing? calculation? This self-appraisal by the patient will largely determine his reactions to the aphasic difficulty and also the personality picture then manifested.

Aphasics cannot be classified by personality patterns because they do not have typical or identical personality aberrations. One aphasic will withdraw completely from social contacts and try to lead a secluded life (due to inability to communicate properly with his environment). The next aphasic may do exactly the opposite. Some aphasics who were thoroughly introverted prior to illness tend to become childishly exhibitionistic following cerebral insult.

After a traumatic onset the aphasic's physical reactions to social situations are usually superior to his language responses. For example, one patient busied with the production of movies prior to illness retained a strong interest in those activities after the onset of aphasia. Unable to participate actively at the studio in making the productions, he derived great pleasure in witnessing those activities. A housewife patient named Sadie evidenced much greater satisfaction in her homemaking endeavors after traumatic onset. One of her last gestures before leaving the clinic was to bake a fruitcake for the staff. These increased interests in homemaking proved most helpful in motivating Sadie's recovery.

However, it is interesting to note that aphasics usually retain much the same basic attitudes about and toward social courtesies as those held prior to illness. Patient Eldon, the "Prince Albert" personality type prior to insult, did not alter his overly attentive attitudes and efforts to observe the usual social graces. Particularly eager for the woman therapist to step into the consulting room ahead of him, Eldon would become greatly disturbed when she failed to comply with his wishes.

Outwardly many aphasics seem to fail in meeting social situations, not because they don't wish to respond properly or as they may have done premorbidly but because they lack communicative abilities. This is especially noticeable when a "global aphasic" (the aphasic who has no speech) is introduced to someone. He may bow and even shake hands but harassment can be discerned in his facial expressions and his physical attitudes. Again, we wish to emphasize that just because one aphasic makes certain social responses (or fails to make them), it will not follow that the next aphasic will duplicate the performance. Each aphasic is an individual who responds to stimuli according to his personal heredity, environmental background, education, life experiences, his physiological and psychological problems, and his present situation.

When considering psychological symptoms it is essential for the therapist to get a clear-cut picture of the aphasic's personality. That means that one must first gather all possible information regarding the life background and the premorbid pattern of this patient's personality. This data usually must be obtained from the patient's relatives or friends and the referring physician because the therapist probably will not have known this aphasic prior to insult. In addition, the therapist should question the nurse and the immediate family as to how the patient is reacting to present hospital or home surroundings. As he works with the patient the therapist will be able to make additional observations. Again, let it be emphasized that every aphasic is an individual! His reactions to the postmorbid environment will reveal his adjustment to psychological and physiological problems arising out of present internal and external stresses, which in turn are influenced by his premorbid personality patterns. Only by keeping all these factors in mind can the therapist devise plans for therapy. In addition, careful note should be made of the behavioral symptoms listed below which experience has taught us to anticipate:

1. Is there any apparent deterioration of mental alertness, memory, and/or association of ideas?
2. Does patient show lack of concentration and shortened auditory memory span?
3. Does he have difficulty in comprehending and sizing up a total situation?
4. Is it difficult for him to meet social situations?
5. How is he adjusting to life situations?
6. Is there reduced ability to discriminate between essential and superficial likenesses?

7. Can he differentiate between essential and unessential details?
8. What ability has he to evaluate past experiences?
9. Does he think only in concrete terms?
10. Is there automatic verbalization?
11. Does he perseverate?
12. Does he lack spontaneity, self-confidence, initiative, and drive?
13. Are there marked attitudes of shyness, seclusiveness, social withdrawal, or impulsiveness?
14. Is there a lack of conformity in thought and behavior?
15. Is he interested in his environment?
16. Can he make any self-appraisal?
17. Is he alert to his environment?
18. Is he irritable?
19. Does he display infantile behavior?
20. Is he easily discouraged?
21. What emotional instability is apparent? Does he cry easily? Or does he suddenly display anger without apparent reasons?
22. Does he express feelings of fear, tension, or anxiety? How?
23. Does he tire quickly? What reason does *he* give for this?
24. Is he cooperative? Uncooperative? Does he give any reason for either attitude?
25. Does he quickly show catastrophic reactions? What seems to start them?
26. Is there euphoria (lack of concern over present disability)?
27. Is there any evidence of psychosis? (Illusions? Hallucinations? Delusions? Suicidal tendencies? Schizophrenia? Paranoia?)
28. Has he had any convulsive seizures since the cerebral insult? How many? What happened?

Every detail of premorbid and postmorbid personality data (together with all present speech and language symptomatology) is extremely useful to the therapist when devising means for preparing and motivating the aphasic's therapy program which will always vary in some ways from the program used with every other patient. See Chapters VII, VIII, and IX for an elaboration.

C. Speech and Language Symptomatology

1. *Receptive Aphasia*

I. *Definition:* A disturbance of perception and/or recognition of noises or sounds (e.g., automobile horn, train whistle, cry of baby, etc.), and/or visible and audible symbols (written or spoken), and a disturbance of recognition and/or significance of animate or inanimate objects. When patients were unable to recognize what was seen, heard, or touched, Jackson termed such impairments of identification as imperception.[12]

II. *Types of Receptive Aphasia:*

A. *Agnosia:* A type of receptive aphasia in which patient lacks ability to recognize and understand written or spoken words, noises, physical activities, and animate or inanimate objects. It is not unusual for a patient to recognize animate objects but be unable to discern inanimate ones, and vice versa. The agnosic may clearly perceive an object, physical activities, or words with his eyes, ears, or sense of touch yet they have no significance to him. Such impairment caused by a disturbance of recognition through one sense organ only is known as *agnosia*.

There are six types of agnosia which pertain particularly to speech and language disturbances: visual ag-

[12] Head, H.: *op. cit.*, p. 26.

nosia, auditory agnosia, music agnosia, tactile agnosia, body agnosia, and agnosia for time and space.

1. *Visual Agnosia:* A disturbance in recognizing objects or physical activities or visible symbols (written words or printed matter) though they may be clearly perceived; an impairment in visual imagination or memory. A patient may see the object or symbol clearly but does not comprehend *what* he has seen. Similarly, a patient may clearly see the *individual* visible letters in the word *dog*, that is *d-o-g*, but fail to understand the word's meaning. Such difficulty is termed *visual agnosia*, or *visual word agnosia*; inability to recognize or differentiate between colors (when there is no existence of color blindness) is *visual color agnosia*; inability to recognize written or printed numbers is *visual number agnosia.*

It should be noted that impairment in recognition may be caused by hysterical amblyopia, a unilateral or bilateral homonymous hemianopia, or by a defect in visual fields. Because of possible problems in the peripheral visual mechanism, such possibilities should be ruled out *before* reaching a diagnosis in the realm of visual agnosia.

Again, a patient may be unable to recognize the letters in the word *dog* because these appear distorted. This recognition loss is due to inability to observe, follow, or re-create lines, figures, or symbols (e.g., circles, squares, triangles) with motoric activity of the eyes, head, or hands. The patient who cannot recognize objects or written or printed word symbols because of loss of the geometric-optic sense (sense of form or direction) has a visual agnosic problem of perception more specifically termed *visual form agnosia* or *geometric-optic agnosia.*

a. *Physiological background:* Various areas of the cortex differ in importance in a particular function and the location of the brain damage usually determines the way in which functional disturbances are revealed. Nielsen[13] found that the area of the cortex necessary for recognition of objects, visible physical activities (running, jumping, etc.), or written or printed words is the convex occipital and parieto-occipital cortex. Loss of ability to recognize numbers is attributed to a lesion of the parietal lobe.

b. *Symptoms:* The recognition loss may precipitate certain associating symptoms:

1ª. *Primary alexia* (also called *agnosic* or *pure alexia*) is an impairment in reading: a disturbance in recognition of visual materials, e.g., letters, figures, syllables, or words, though these may be clearly perceived with the peripheral visual mechanism.

Sometimes reading ability is entirely lost because the patient has lost his ability in visual imagery. Reading ability may be only partially lost according to the nature and extent of brain injury.

a¹. Patient may have normal visual acuity for simply formed letters such as *O, C, I*, etc., but cannot recognize complicated ones such as *H, A, R*, etc. This disturbs his reading ability.

b¹. Patient may have normal visual recognition but cannot discern the form of the simplest letters, e.g., *O, C, I*, etc.

c¹. Patient may be unable to read letters but

[13] Nielsen, J. M.: *Agnosia, Apraxia, Aphasia*, 2nd ed. Paul B. Hoeber, Inc., New York, 1946, pp. 252, 264.

can read numbers. For example, although surgeon-patient Dr. B. was unable to read most words, he could recognize the figures on the stock market page; numbers seemed to be "concrete" objects to him.

d¹. In less serious disturbances of visual recognition, the patient may read with understanding simple phrases or statements involving only a few words, but reading complicated statements is impossible. Nielsen described these alexic problems as *semantic alexia*. Loss of ability to recognize letters, figures, words, he termed *agnosic alexia*.

e¹. In extreme cases, a patient cannot read numbers nor do written calculations. Inability to read numbers is termed *visual number agnosia* or *mathematical alexia* (see page 22). When agnosia problems occur in conjunction with inability to calculate, the disturbance is known as *acalculia*. The patient who has not lost the meaning of numbers may be able to do oral mathematical problems. If premorbidly he "whispered" or talked to himself while making written calculations, most likely the ability to make written calculations will remain intact. Sometimes a patient can utter numbers in series but lacks all concept as to their meaning or values.

f¹. Patient may have *completely* lost the ability of visual recognition. This problem is a severe form of primary alexia.

2ª. *Paraphasia:* A disturbance in diction, and/or

grammar, and/or syntax which may show up as a distortion in writing; a distortion in the oral formulation of sounds or words; in the substitution of sounds or words; and in misplacement or omission of sounds, syllables, or words. There are three types of paraphasia:

a¹. *Paragrammatism:* That type of paraphasia manifested by:

1ᵇ. Omission of sounds or syllables within the word.

2ᵇ. Reversal of sounds or syllables within the word. Sounds are not marshaled in accurate sequences.

3ᵇ. Substitution of sounds or syllables within the word.

4ᵇ. Syllables may be substituted, omitted, or reversed within a word. Prefixes and suffixes are usually the syllables most disturbed.

5ᵇ. Reversal of words in a sentence. Circumlocutions are used to avoid saying "difficult" words. In certain instances a stutter may be manifested.

6ᵇ. Practically unintelligible speech. Words are garbled and speech is confused or divorced from thought. Such language has been characterized as *"jargon" aphasia.* Head referred to this problem as *syntactical aphasia;* Kussmaul spoke of it as *choreatic aphasia;* Pick described it as *cataphasia,* referring to all three problems of disturbance in grammar, syntax, and diction.

        7[b]. Paragrammatism appears more often in receptive aphasia than does agrammatism.

  b[1]. *Agrammatism:* A type of paraphasia manifested most frequently within a sentence by:

        1[b]. Omission of grammatical words to such an extent that the speech may be described as telegram style. Omitted words are not necessarily motorically difficult and may not be needed to supply the meaning of the sentence.

        Prepositions, conjunctions, and articles such as *in, on, to, up, and, but, a, the* are usually omitted. If used, they are generally employed erroneously.

        2[b]. Sentences may be shortened or reversed in form.

        3[b]. The thought process loses its aim, is unable to reach its original goal, and results in a "word-salad." Thus words are replaced by others incidentally associated in the mind of the patient. For example, formerly loquacious and glib, patient John would remark: "As though I might look at something with same weight. I have it forward. It has a long weight. I have nothing to go to. It might be fingers—or standard of anything. I lick from anything." Fully aware that much of his voluble language is not understandable to his listener, it does not seem to disturb him. Often he seems entirely unaware of these errors.

4^b. Some sounds may be omitted or substituted though patient may have no
motoric problems in producing them.
Jane says, "I was ma ands soap" for "I
wash my hand with soap." Also, she
says *sace* when she means to say *face*;
was for *wash*; *moder* for *mother*. John
says *me* for *my*, *mees* for *knees*, *mose*
for *nose*.

5^b. Agrammatism appears in some cases
of receptive aphasia but most often in
cases of expressive aphasia. (See Expressive Aphasia, page 37.)

c¹. *Mixed paraphasia:* A type of paraphasia
which exhibits problems of paragramma-
tism and of agrammatism. Goldstein referred to this as "abstract-attitude" paraphasia. Apparently he used this terminology because the patient is deficient in
abstract attitude.

1^b. *Physiological background:* Goldstein
observed that this type of paraphasia
occurs in patients with sensory or
motor aphasia where "the lesion does
not affect the motor or sensory part of
the speech area alone, but also the area
important for inner speech."[14]

2^b. *Symptoms:*

a². Characteristic hesitation of speech
as found in agrammatism is not
present.

b². Substitution of one word for another with the substituted word

---

[14] Goldstein, Kurt: *Language and Language Disturbances.* Grune & Stratton,
Inc., New York, 1948, p. 84.

usually somewhat related to the
correct one.

c^2. Reversal of sounds or syllables
within a word although the sounds
may not be motorically distorted.

d^2. Omission or reversal of sounds or
syllables within a word. This problem is not exhibited much in the
utterance of word series and motor
speech patterns.

e^2. Misplacement of accent within a
word.

f^2. Rhythm of word is distorted.

3^a. *Paragraphia:*

a^1. In severe cases of primary alexia the patient may be unable to write a word (i.e.,
agraphia) because he cannot recall what
the word "looks like." He is disturbed in
writing because of this problem in visual
verbal recall (i.e., in remembering how
the letters are formed, the order of the letters in the word, etc.)

b^1. Where there is a complete loss of visual
recognition, it is usually impossible for the
patient to copy the simplest written or
printed matter.

c^1. Some visual agnosics cannot recognize
geometric forms and are unable to distinguish between height and width. (See
page 22.) The paragraphia then creates
difficulty in forming letters because these
patients cannot recognize accurately how
the letters should be made.

d^1. The paraphasic has difficulty in formulating words and language and in writing

words. He omits letters or words or reverses syllables or changes the order of letters. Consonants may be substituted. The
writing difficulties usually mirror his
speech defect. (See Paraphasia, page 24.)
In such a case, the problem would be a secondary agraphia because it would be mir-
roring the aphasic difficulty.

e[1]. Later it will be noted that paragraphia
may result from difficulties in auditory
verbal recall or from damage to the motor
(writing) area. (See Auditory Agnosia,
page 30.)

4[a]. *Dysarthria* (central in origin) is common to
various aphasics and frequently occurs in
nonaphasics. This central type of dysarthria
appears as an associating symptom to the
aphasia.

Because of sluggish tongue functioning, the
"central" dysarthric patient has difficulty
moving that organ from one position to another. He is handicapped in making rhythmic
repetitive movements with it. Some aphasics
find it difficult to produce any tongue movements at all. The patient manifests the following symptoms:

a[1]. Articulates incorrectly the consonant
sounds.

b[1]. Omits consonants of a word as he attempts
to utter subsequent words of the sentence.

c[1]. Elides consonants to the point where his
speech sounds are "sloppy."

d[1]. Substitutes consonant sounds.

e[1]. Reverses the order of consonants within a
sentence.

f^1. Spasmodic interruptions in utterance.

g^1. Sudden increases and decreases in volume.

2. *Auditory Agnosia:* A type of receptive aphasia manifested by the patient's imperception of the meaning of audible sounds or spoken words (though his peripheral auditory mechanism and his eighth cranial nerve are intact). He cannot understand oral language although clearly hearing the spoken words. Marked auditory agnosia is not frequently observed. However, auditory agnosia in the mild form is a common symptom among aphasics. Authorities have used other terms for this such as *acoustic agnosia, cortical sensory aphasia, psychic deafness, Wernicke's aphasia,* and *word deafness.* Inability to understand oral words is termed *auditory verbal agnosia.* Inability to understand oral numbers is *auditory number agnosia.*

a. *Physiological background:* The lesion may be in the superior convolution of the temporal lobe. A lesion in the posterior part of the superior temporal gyrus also may produce auditory aphasia with all its concomitants.

While it requires only a very delicate lesion in the temporal lobe to produce a subcortical sensory aphasia, nevertheless Goldstein in *Aftereffects of Brain Injuries in War* declared that subcortical sensory aphasia (*pure word deafness, pure speech deafness,* or *peripheral sensory aphasia*) never has been observed so far as he knew. He felt this was understandable when one considers the "very circumscribed delicate lesion in the temporal lobe necessary to produce this form of aphasia."[15] In

---

[15] Goldstein, Kurt: *Aftereffects of Brain Injuries in War.* Grune & Stratton, Inc., New York, 1942, p. 163.

his later book, *Language and Language Disturbances*, he observed that *pure word deafness* (peripheral sensory aphasia) was due to an "incomplete damage of the area of acoustic perception which does not disturb acoustic perception in general, but dedifferentiates more or less the complex acoustic phenomena which correspond to language (acoustic speech *Gestalten*)."[16] The patient cannot understand anything he hears. But reading, writing, and oral speech are intact. However, oral speech sounds like some foreign language to him. When the lesion in the temporal lobe is somewhat more extensive, *auditory agnosia*, i.e., *cortical sensory aphasia* or *word deafness*, may be manifested while in other patients a more or less *general deafness* would occur. Hearing problems frequently result from gunshot injury and auditory agnosia often occurs in combination with visual agnosia.

b. *Symptoms:* Just as a person may have imperception in the visual realm, this recognition disturbance may also occur in the realm of hearing. For instance, a patient with a normal ear mechanism may hear the sound of a dog barking but be unaware that the sound heard is a bark. He may hear the utterance of the word *dog* and still not get any meaning from that word.

1ª. Patient does not understand what he hears. He may know words are being spoken but they have no meaning for him.

2ª. Patient has shortened auditory memory span, a problem evidenced even in the mildest cases of auditory agnosia.

---

[16] Goldstein, Kurt: *Language and Language Disturbances.* Grune & Stratton, Inc., New York, 1948, p. 221.

3ᵃ. Patient may understand short, simple sentences but cannot understand longer sentences.

4ᵃ. He may comprehend simple directions but flounder when given complicated or involved commands.

5ᵃ. He has difficulty in repetition of language said to him.

6ᵃ. Paraphasia is evidenced. (See pages 24–26.)

7ᵃ. He has difficulty in writing—*paragraphia*.

   a¹. Because of inability to understand the language he hears, patient is deficient in writing from dictation. Not comprehending the dictated word, he is handicapped in writing it. Hence his writing deficiency corresponds to the speech disturbance.

   b¹. Difficulty in writing may also result from inability to remember "how the word sounds." Unable to recall the concept of the spoken word, he is handicapped in writing it.

   c¹. Paragraphia may result from difficulty in formulating language (i.e., his paraphasic problem).

3. *Music Agnosia* (also called *amusia*): A disturbance in the recognition of music. Two types are recognized:

   a. *Visual music agnosia:* Difficulty in recognizing visual music symbols.

      1ᵃ. *Physiological background:* Nielsen[17] observed that visual music agnosia is caused by a lesion of the occipital lobe and that impulses from both *ariae striatae* do not reach the angular

[17] Nielsen, J. M.: *op. cit.*, p. 261.

gyrus for recognition. In such cases usually there is an associated homonymous hemianopia.

2ª. *Symptoms:* Inability to read musical notes.

b. *Auditory music agnosia:* Difficulty in recognizing musical sounds—vocal or instrumental.

1ª. *Physiological background:* Auditory music agnosia results from extensive damage to the connections of the transverse temporal cortex.

2ª. Patients may be unable to:

a¹. Recognize musical notes or remember music.

b¹. Distinguish between various musical selections.

c¹. Differentiate the sound of one musical instrument from that of another.

d¹. Distinguish differences of pitch, inflection, and volume.

e¹. Comprehend the mood expressed in the music.

4. *Tactile Agnosia:* A disturbance in recognizing objects through the sense of feeling or touch. For instance, patient may handle a piece of cotton or silk or wood, etc., but not know what he is feeling.

Similarly, patient may disclose tactile difficulty by inability to recognize an object from its form when he touches or handles it. This is termed *astereognosis* (also called stereoagnosis). He may describe the form or shape of an object adequately but fail to grasp the symbolic meaning of what he is describing.

a. *Physiological background:* Tactile agnosia appears as a result of lesions of the parietal lobe, posterior to the posterior central convolution.

Krueger[18] observed astereognosis in the parietal lobe. Foerster[19] also noted astereognosis resulting from lesions of the posterior central convolution.

  b. *Symptoms:*
    1[a]. Difficulty in recognizing material out of which an object is made (e.g., wood, glass, wool, silk, etc.).
    2[a]. Difficulty in recognizing objects by shape or form (astereognosis).

5. *Body Agnosia* (*autotopagnosia* or *topagnosia*): A disturbance in ability to recognize or localize various parts of the body. Difficulty in recognizing the fingers is called *finger agnosia*.

  a. *Physiological background:* Body agnosia is not localized on the basis of present known material. Muncie[20] suggested that it probably results from lesions of the posterior portion of the parietal lobe. Finger agnosia seems to be caused by lesions in the supramarginal gyrus.

  b. *Symptoms:*
    1[a]. Patient may be unable to recognize various parts of his body. Asked to point to his arm, he may place his hand on his knee.
    2[a]. Patient may lose a body part and deny its loss, a problem first described by Charcot.
    3[a]. Patient may skilfully use his hand but cannot name or designate, on command, the various fingers (finger agnosia).

6. *Agnosia for Time and Space:* A disturbance in orientation manifested by inability to tell time, to

[18] Krueger, J.: "Ueber Sensibilitaetsstoerungen nach Verletzungen der Grosshirnrinde," *Ztschr. f. d. ges. Neurol. u. Psychiat.*, 33:74, 1916.

[19] Foerster, O.: "Die Topik der Sensibilitaetsstoerungen bei Unterbrechung der Sensiblen Leitungsbahnen," *Neurol. Zentralbl.*, 35:807, 1916.

[20] Muncie, Wendell: *Psychobiology and Psychiatry*, 2nd ed. C. V. Mosby Co., St. Louis, 1948, p. 483.

judge space and distance, or differentiate between right and left.

    a. *Physiological background:* Bonhoeffer[21] attributed localization of agnosia for time and space to the angular gyrus.

    b. Patient may be unable to:

        1[a]. Differentiate between the left and right side of his body. This may exist independently of body agnosia but frequently occurs concurrently.

        2[a]. Differentiate between *above, below; in front, behind; up, down.*

        3[a]. Follow directions to a given geographic goal.

        4[a]. Point out familiar places on a map.

        5[a]. Judge passage of time or tell time by looking at the clock.

B. *Transcortical Sensory Aphasia* (termed central sensory aphasia by Goldstein): A type manifested by patient's ability to repeat whatever is asked of him though he does not understand it. His problem is partly expressive and partly receptive.

    1. *Physiological background:* Nielsen[22] stated that in transcortical sensory aphasia, the lesion "affects the Wernicke's area or a short portion of the cortex between it and the angular gyrus." Goldstein[23] felt the temporal lobe must be affected but without damage to the acoustic area. He noted that transcortical sensory aphasia can occur in a state of restitution of Wernicke's aphasia.

    2. *Symptoms:*

        a. Though patient fails to understand something said to him, he can repeat it in correct motoric

---

[21] *Ibid.*, p. 483.

[22] Nielsen, J. M.: *op. cit.*, p. 267.

[23] Goldstein, Kurt: *Language and Language Disturbances.* Grune & Stratton, Inc., New York, 1948, p. 298.

language. Sometimes he may repeat automatically and compulsively (i.e., echolalia) without comprehension. Again, as he repeats material, it may become meaningful to him. He may repeat over and over, finally stopping when his speech is scarcely audible. Some repeat for hours, which (psychologically) is a reversion to infantile attitudes. Normal children often manifest oral echolalia as a form of exhibitionism.

b. Spontaneous speech may be disturbed but usually the ability to understand is more seriously affected than spontaneous speech.

c. Patient tends to speak a great deal but has difficulty in perceiving words, phrases, or sentences as complete wholes.

d. Due to impaired abstract attitude, patient may be so disturbed in understanding spontaneous speech as to refrain from speaking through fear of making errors.

e. Paraphasia:

1a. Sounds in a word may be omitted.

2a. Sounds of words may be changed in order.

3a. First sound or sounds of word may be correct; then there may be remnant final sounds. Or last part of word may be entirely absent.

4a. Sounds in center of word may be omitted.

5a. Part of word may not be marshaled in correct sequence.

6a. Word may retain its previous rhythm and length but some prominent sound or sounds may be omitted.

f. If wrong words (in meaning) are used, usually they exhibit little or no paraphasia.

g. Circumlocutions are not used as often as in the case of the amnesic aphasic.

h. Patient can start a word or number series on command without having to be given a key sound or initial member of the series.

i. What he is able to read accurately usually is not comprehended.

j. Patient's ability to produce spontaneous speech and to repeat is more disturbed than his ability to understand.

k. Patient is usually rather voluble in speaking.

l. Paragraphia is frequently one of the first disturbances to appear.

   1ª. Patient is unable to write spontaneously.

   2ª. The writing deficiency corresponds to the speech disturbance.

   3ª. Spontaneous writing is somewhat more disturbed than spontaneous speaking.

2. *Expressive Aphasia*

I. *Definition:* A disturbance of symbolization which alters the normal visible or audible production of one's ideas. This is the type most frequently encountered by therapists because it involves the frontal part of Broca's area, which is particularly vulnerable to lesions from violence.

II. *Types of Expressive Aphasia:*

A. *Apraxia* is a disturbance in ability to perform a specific requested or desired motor act. Patient may not exhibit any evidence of paresis but seems utterly unable to act motorically or to marshal and guide the muscle groups involved. He may know what he wants to say or do but cannot cause the muscles to perform the desired functions. His motor speech patterns (as well as other motor patterns) are disturbed and the resulting phenomenon is termed apraxia.

1. *Physiological background:* Sittig and Mingazzini

asserted that apraxia resulted from lesions in the corpus callosum, but Liepmann found apraxia present when the areas particularly involved were the left parietal lobe, the precentral gyrus, the parieto-occipital region, and the corpus callosum. He claimed, furthermore, that the "practice function of the right precentral gyrus was not subject to the person's will without guidance through the left precentral gyrus, and that any lesion of the major side caused apraxia of both sides."[24] Nielsen[25] made similar findings but declared the right side is merely untrained and that after a lesion of the major side, the minor one soon develops its function unless a progressive lesion is present.

2. *Symptoms:*

  a. Patient has difficulty in word-naming.

  b. He may express an idea, e.g., *apple*, but in motorically defective, garbled speech. The impairment arises from inability to think of the idea of *apple* long enough to express it correctly in motoric speech.

  c. Similarly, he may formulate ideas for a plan of action but can't retain the ideas sufficiently long to carry them out. He may even do something opposite to his own desires, thus appearing to be absent-minded. Some writers call this *ideational apraxia.* John (a patient) placed the wrong end of a cork-tipped cigarette in his mouth when starting to smoke. Bill frequently tries to write with the wrong end of a pencil. Jack starts to write with his index finger rather than with the pencil.

---

[24] Liepmann, H.: "Das Krankheitsbild der Apraxia (motorische Asymbolie)," *Monatschr. f. Psychiat. u. Neurol.*, Vol. 8, 1900.
[25] Nielsen, J. M.: *op. cit.*, p. 59.

Patient may utilize speech muscles to utter something contrary to what he wished. For instance, he may wish to say *dog* but utters *cat*. Jane may want to say "I wash my *hands*" but says "I wash my *face*." This utterance of incorrect words usually causes frustration.

d. When a request or command is made by audible or visible symbols (either oral or pantomimic), patient is unable to comply. For example, with apraxia of the hand muscles he cannot light a match, cut with scissors, or grasp silverware, pencils, etc.; with construction apraxia, patient can grasp an object but cannot use the hands in a planned activity. Prior to trauma patient Judy was an accomplished seamstress skilfully handling needle, thread, and scissors, but she entirely lost the ability to cut out a dress and sew it together.

With apraxia of the speech muscles, patient cannot mimic such acts as biting the lips, smacking the lips, whistling, protruding the tongue, wiping the lips with the tongue, etc. Shown an object, he cannot grasp the idea of it. He may fail to copy or write *what the object is* from dictation. (However, these patients often can write the *word* from dictation.) He may see or hear an act performed (e.g., running, singing, etc.) but cannot write the name of the act. The difficulty is termed *ideokinetic apraxia*.

Patient may lose all ability to use speech muscles. He may mentally retain adequate visible and audible symbols but cannot marshal and guide the speech muscles to form words. On request he may protrude the tongue or use the mouth muscles to form words he wants to say, yet oral speech is impossible.

e. Certain associative symptoms sometime appear with apraxia of the speech muscles:

1ª. Patient's paraphasia may create disturbance in diction, grammar, syntax, or all of these. This is manifested by *paragrammatism* and *agrammatism*.

a¹. Paragrammatism: (See pages 25–26.)

1ᵇ. Words may be omitted.

2ᵇ. Sounds may be substituted.

3ᵇ. Sounds may be reversed or misplaced within a word.

4ᵇ. Words may be reversed in a sentence.

b¹. Agrammatism: (See pages 26–27.)

1ᵇ. There may be lack of fluency in speaking or speech may be slow because of patient's difficulty in selecting correct grammatical forms such as articles, prepositions, prefixes, suffixes, auxiliary verbs, etc. He may use the simplest forms, e.g., infinitives.

2ᵇ. He may have difficulty in saying words in a series.

3ᵇ. There may be omission of grammatical words to such an extent that speech may be of telegram style.

2ª. Patient frequently can recite words in series but will fail to produce them in isolation. By reciting the series, he can stop to utter the one desired; i.e., the word can be said better in series than when spoken alone. Often he pronounces correctly in a song some word he cannot say in isolated oral speech. When patient Jack sings "Over There," he accurately utters the words *over there* and *everywhere* but saying them in isolation is difficult and at times almost impossible.

3[a]. Patient may have difficulty reciting numbers in series. He may not be able to recite the multiplication tables or to count by 2's, 4's, 6's, etc. Disturbance in the ability to calculate often occurs in apraxia involving speech musculature.

4[a]. Patient may recognize numbers shown to him but cannot name them.

5[a]. Patient may be unable to write individual numbers correctly.

6[a]. Patient may be unable to write digits in series or to give you his address, telephone number, the day of the week, the date, etc.

7[a]. Patient may handle numbers from 1 to 25 but cannot use higher numbers.

8[a]. Patient may use lower numbers related to concrete acts or objects such as paying carfare, buying small articles in a dime store (articles costing 25 cents or less) but cannot handle small numbers when adding, subtracting, dividing, or multiplying. This may be due to inability to perform abstract thinking.

9[a]. When unable to count in series or write specific digits, etc., as explained under items 4[a], 5[a], 6[a], and 7[a] above, patient's ability to calculate is always disturbed. This problem of dealing with small numbers is known as *low-level number apraxia*; difficulty in calculation is termed *acalculia* or *calculation apraxia*. However, the patient with acalculia is not necessarily disturbed in handling lower level numbers and may be able to count in series, write digits, etc.

10ᵃ. Patient may use speech musculature for all purposes except speech yet present speech and language symptoms similar to those in patients *unable* to use the speech musculature for all purposes. (See point *d*, pages 39–40.)

11ᵃ. Patient may have difficulty in writing— *apractic agraphia.*

 aᵃ. Patient may be unable to write because he cannot hold a pencil or pen. This creates such anxiety that he feels frustrated or even overtly angry, displaying flurries of temper. Patient Pauline tends to grasp a pencil as though holding a baseball bat. When she attempts to hold the pencil normally, she becomes emotionally upset and frequently cries.

 bᵃ. Patient's difficulty in writing or forming letters and words correctly may be caused by inability to coordinate the preferred hand for writing or there may be hemiplegia of the dominant side and the "writing hand" is paralyzed. These patients must be trained through the nondominant hand. Under the discussion of therapy, pages 137–39, it will be seen that the problem of writing should be attacked in the initial stages of the therapeutic program. Some workers in the aphasia field are of the opinion that writing should always be attacked as a separate training goal, but our experience contraindicates this. We have found that writing can best be molded and developed along with the speech and language therapy. For a discussion of this aspect of therapy, see pages 110–12.

c¹. Patient may be unable to differentiate between certain letters. Patient Bill frequently writes *f* when he means *p*; *o* when he intends to write *a*; *e* for *i*; and often fails to notice the difference between incorrect letters. However, he can write his own name because that is one of *his* fixed "retrained" motor patterns. Bill has similar difficulty in drawing other object forms.

d¹. Patient may be unable to form letters properly, making wrong hooks. Patient Bill confuses *g* with *q* and frequently ponders over the form of a letter before producing it. Sometimes he writes a letter incorrectly but usually recognizes the error.

e¹. Patient may be disturbed in ability to copy, to write spontaneously, or to write from dictation.

12ᵃ. Patient may have difficulty in using his hands for various aspects of construction or manipulation (*construction apraxia*). A musician patient may be unable to play an instrument. We had a professional cornetist (a white male, aged 62) who lost the ability to use his instrument although he could read musical signs. (See Visual Music Agnosia, pages 32–33.) Patient Ed, a draftsman, lost the ability to make intricate drawings. Patient Bob, a surgeon, forgot how to proceed sequentially when performing an operation. Patient Al, a carpenter, forgot how to use tools in building a structure. Such loss is always upsetting and more or less frustrating in any patient whose premorbid history indicates a real interest in handicraft. The patient may be able to hold and move an instrument or tool, but the loss of digital and manual skill usually arouses grief.

f. When patient exhibits apraxia in the writing realm only, the difficulty is termed *isolated agraphia*, revealed by the inability to marshal and guide hand movements for writing, although the same muscle groups involved may be used adequately for other purposes. Isolated agraphia may also result from a lesion of the writing center at the foot of the second frontal convolution, but such patients cannot write with hand movements and usually find it impossible to type words or spell them with blocks. Patients harassed by these inadequacies often experience catastrophic reactions.

g. Apraxia may occur in conjunction with pure motor aphasia. The symptoms are determined by (1^a) nature and extent of the cerebral insult, and (2^a) the patient's premorbid organization of speech patterns and the nature of the damage postmorbidly.

B. *Pure motor aphasia* (by Goldstein termed *peripheral motor aphasia*, but called *verbal aphasia* by Head) is characterized by loss of spontaneous speech without relative deterioration of intelligence or ability to think in abstractions.

1. *Physiological background:* Some authorities speak of pure motor aphasia as *Broca's aphasia* because the disturbance is produced by a lesion in Broca's area. The causative lesion occurs in the cortex of the left

third convolution but may extend into neighboring areas of the frontal lobe and into the insula.

Nielsen's[26] findings indicate that the lesion causing pure motor aphasia is usually traumatic or vascular. The cortex or subcortex at the foot of the third frontal convolution of the major side is affected. Nielsen analyzed further the physiological aspect of pure motor aphasia by explaining that the emissive speech evidenced after a disturbance of Broca's area is due to training in the corresponding area of the other hemisphere. He also observed that language remaining after a cerebral injury is determined by the undamaged remaining language mechanism. Should aphasia appear, there is either no performance in the sphere of function under consideration or there is faulty performance. In either case, the major cerebral hemisphere is affected. Absence of performance means that neither hemisphere is functioning; faulty performance means that the minor hemisphere is working imperfectly.

The left side of the cortex is usully the major side, although pure motor aphasia has been observed in patients whose right hemisphere was dominant.

Goldstein[27] in *Language and Language Disturbances* made similar observations. He pointed out that an occasional individual suffering extensive lesions of the left Broca's area did not have a motor aphasia. Where aphasia was present initially, good language returns rapidly and without any special practices or exercises. He assumed the left area of Broca in these patients had cooperated closely with the corresponding area in the right hemisphere.

[26] *Ibid.*, pp. 66, 93–137.
[27] Goldstein, Kurt: *Language and Language Disturbances.* Grune & Stratton, Inc., New York, 1948, pp. 204–5.

However, he insisted that all connections through the corpus callosum between the operculum Rolandi and the central speech mechanisms of both hemispheres must be preserved in order to activate the Broca's area of the right hemisphere.

Goldstein further noticed that there could be large lesions in the left Broca's area along with manifestations of motor aphasia. These cases improved markedly with exercises but otherwise did not progress satisfactorily. He felt advancement in such cases could not be considered as new learning accomplished through the aid of the other hemisphere, but rather as improvement through the effect of speech and language exercises which tended to utilize the residual, though defective, areas of the left hemisphere.

He described a third type of patient with complete initial word muteness in which the return of motor speech was gradual and incomplete, even with exercises. He believed this slight speech improvement resulted from a taking-over by the corresponding right area of an activity it had previously shared, and not by restitution of language through any improved function of the left area. He assumed the right area had slowly acquired an entirely new activity. Such cases did not show spontaneous return of speech and the patient seldom regained normal premorbid promptness, even with exercises. Usually this type continued to suffer marked motor difficulties. (For other remarks on this, see Therapeutic Suggestions for Pure Motor Aphasia, pages 153–54.)

2. *Symptoms:*

   a. Immediately after cerebral insult the patient may be speechless or unable to repeat or read aloud. Remaining speech may be limited to the word *no* or may include words like *yes, no, mother,* etc. Sometimes the patient utters swear words unintentionally but is unable to say them on command.

b. Patient usually has a strong desire to express himself although possessing little or no spontaneous speech. Again, he may have a compulsion to utter what he does not wish to say.

c. When there is residual emissive speech, the sounds and words usually are motorically disturbed. As a result of damage to previously acquired motor speech patterns, the pure motor aphasic frequently exhibits apraxic difficulties of the lips and tongue. (See Expressive Aphasia, Apraxia, page 37.) The lips and tongue may be used for eating or the tongue may be protruded reflexly, but the patient cannot employ them motorically for speech.

d. Understanding of oral speech is rapidly regained after cerebral insult.

e. Dysarthria (central in origin): See Dysarthria, page 29.

f. Meaningful words may be incorrectly articulated (due to loss of motoric fluency), but patient's intelligence may show little or no reduction.

g. Patient has difficulty in word-finding because of damage to the instrumentalities of speech (i.e., loss of motoric fluency). Words particularly affected are nouns and verbs, while small words like prepositions and articles are lacking in spontaneous speech.

h. Patient may reacquire ability to utter more and more words but still may articulate incorrectly.

Uttering isolated sounds may be more difficult than enunciating words or sentences.

i. Some patients spontaneously repeat words with less articulation difficulty than when they try to speak on command. However, the motoric difficulty in repetition and spontaneous speech is primarily the same.

j. When patient Margaret is asked to utter a certain word such as *horse*, she says "o." However, repeating it over and over, she usually can come forth with *ho* and sometimes *hor*. The performance is defective because there is no *s*. This difficulty in repetition is typical of pure motor aphasia. Voluntary trial-and-error movements tend to improve performance.

k. It is easier for the patient to repeat words than to say them spontaneously. He may have more difficulty in repeating long words than he does short ones.

l. If the patient utters words in series, e.g., *one*, *two*, *three*, *four*, etc., he may have difficulty in the distortion of sounds in the various words. Patient Grace exerts much effort and perseverance to marshal the number series, 1 to 10.

m. When patient Margaret is given the first word of a number series, e.g., *one*, her performance of the series does not improve. Similarly, given the first sound of a word, her utterance of that word is not facilitated. This is a typical symptom of pure motor aphasia.

n. Patient may give the characteristic consonants or vowels of a specific word but cannot say the word itself. He may also be able to tell if the word is "long" or "short."

o. Paraphasia may be present. As pointed out

earlier (pages 26–27), paraphasia may occur in both expressive aphasia and receptive aphasia.

1ª. *Types of paraphasia:*

    a¹. *Paragrammatism:* As mentioned in the discussion of visual agnosia (page 25), this disturbance is manifested by omission of sounds or syllables within a word, substitution of sounds or syllables within a word, and reversal of words in a sentence. It occurs less often in expressive aphasia than in receptive aphasia.

    b¹. *Agrammatism:* Occurs most often in expressive aphasia, less often in receptive aphasia.

        1ᵇ. *Symptoms:*

            a². Patient may tend to use the simplest types of grammatical forms, e.g., infinitives.

            b². There may be omission of grammatical words to such an extent that the speech may be described as telegram style. Words omitted are not necessarily motorically difficult but are unnecessary to supply meaning to the sentence. However, words may be omitted because they are motorically impeded. Some sounds may be omitted because the patient cannot pronounce them correctly. He occasionally may stop speaking entirely because of emotional disturbance from motor handicaps.

            c². There may be substitution of sounds.

d^2. There may be hesitancies in speech caused by the attempt to speak motorically in a fluent manner.

e^2. There may be distortion of sounds.

f^2. Patient tends to perseverate on other sounds which he can say correctly.

g^2. Patient may tend to reverse or misplace sounds within a word.

p. Reading aloud is disturbed.

1^a. Inability to utter words motorically may prevent patient's reading aloud, yet he reads silently and even comprehends material read. Such oral reading problems are known as *secondary alexia.*

2^a. Patient may tend to omit small words (prepositions and articles) in reading.

3^a. Patient reading aloud may make the same errors as he does in oral speech (i.e., secondary alexia). Often ability to read aloud excels patient's capacity to speak.

q. Writing may be disturbed.

1^a. Sometimes motor paragraphia accompanies pure motor aphasia, probably because the lesion causing pure motor aphasia is so near the area involved in motor paragraphia.

2^a. Paragraphia is sometimes evidenced in pure motor aphasic patients who tend to whisper words as they write. The ability to whisper words is disturbed so the writing is affected.

3^a. Patient may lose ability to write spontaneously or to copy or write from dictation, yet still be able to say and write his name.

4^a. The capacity to write may be restored in much the same manner as speech is regained, but the writing may show paraphasic errors similar to those in oral speech.

5ª. Writing may be somewhat paragraphic, especially agrammatic (typical telegram style).

6ª. Frequently patient writes better from dictation than he writes voluntarily.

7ª. Patient may be able to write some words correctly if the motor writing patterns have not been disturbed.

r. Patient may adequately perform simple arithmetical problems.

s. Some pure motor aphasics manifest associative stuttering symptoms, especially when the patient is truly aware of the full scope of his speech loss. This realization may produce almost an aphonia.

t. Patient may or may not lose the ability to sing. Sometimes he can sing the melody but cannot speak the words. Patient Gladys at first could only hum "Row, row, row your boat." Now she sings the words clearly. Goldstein[28] observed that where singing had been enjoyable and an "emotional outlet" premorbidly, the patient's singing capacity was more disturbed than with a patient whose attitude had been matter-of-fact toward singing. We have observed this occasionally but feel the disturbed attitude has its roots in psychic frustrations as well as in physiological problems.

u. Patient may have difficulty calculating orally. This occurs when patient had memorized the multiplication tables by rote as a motor series. Inability to say the multiplication tables naturally impairs using them to perform calculations.

A patient may be able to handle mathematical problems with paper and pencil, but if he pre-

[28] *Ibid.*, pp. 122–24, 147.

morbidly always whispered what he was writing, the whisper loss will prevent him from making written calculations.

v. If patient premorbidly spoke aloud or whispered when reading, he will have difficulty in reading postmorbidly because he cannot marshal words motorically and it becomes almost impossible for him to understand what he reads. The "feel" and sound of oral speech are needed for full comprehension. This secondary aspect of reading difficulty is termed *secondary alexia.*

C. *Transcortical motor aphasia* is marked by difficulty in word-finding and spontaneous speech even though the patient seems not to have difficulty in abstract attitude nor any general mental impairment.

1. *Physiological background:* Opinion varies as to the etiology of this problem. Some authorities suggest the cause is a partial lesion of the cortex in the region of the posterior part of the third frontal convolution.

Goldstein observed that the cause was usually of a traumatic nature (e.g., brain pressures caused by tumors, abscesses, etc.), and that the disturbance apparently lies between the sensory and motor area; hence the name *transcortical motor aphasia.* Nielsen noted that transcortical motor aphasia was "due to lesions which in others would cause Broca's aphasia, but a good power of initiation of speech is present through stimulation by the spoken word of the examiner, of Wernicke's area."[29]

2. *Symptoms:*

a. Patient has difficulty in word-finding although he can think abstractly, i.e., assume an abstract attitude.

b. Patient's understanding of speech may be im-

[29] Nielsen, J. M.: *op. cit.,* pp. 66–67.

paired enough to make him unable to comprehend accurately what a word means when he hears it.

c. Patient has no marked problem in uttering words volitionally, but perseverance on his part fails to improve his speech.

d. Whatever speech (spontaneous or repetitious) he produces has few or no motoric defects.

e. Patient may repeat words more easily than he can utter them in voluntary spontaneous speech.

f. He may repeat sounds or words which he cannot say volitionally or on command. Also, he can repeat accurately words and sentences he has just heard but will fail to comprehend what he uttered. Speech tends to be "automatic."

g. Patient repeats what is requested although not repeating the words as he hears them (as in the case of true echolalia). Instead, he selects the correct answer. When patient Bill was asked, "Can you say *Los Angeles?*" he did not make the typical echolalic reply of "Can you say *Los Angeles?*" but answered *"Los Angeles,"* revealing selective ability.

h. Patient has difficulty in uttering words in series but discloses no motor speech error. Giving the first sound or word of a series of words or numbers may stimulate patient to proceed with the series, yet this perseverance is of little or no help to him even though he may make conscious efforts in word-finding.

i. Patient reads aloud better than in spontaneous speech. Reading aloud is sometimes better than repetition.

j. Patient's ability to repeat is somewhat commensurate with his ability to read.

    k. Patient may evidence difficulty in writing.

        1ᵃ. He may copy mechanically and write from dictation but sometimes is disturbed by the effort. He may write part of a word but cannot complete it. The impulse is not adequate to produce the entire word.

        2ᵃ. He may reveal loss of ability to write spontaneously.

        3ᵃ. There may be motor agrammatism evidenced by patient's difficulty in finding grammatical forms. He may select the simplest types, e.g., infinitives.

D. *Central motor aphasia* is a form of expressive aphasia in which the patient has neuromotor difficulty in speaking spontaneously and reading aloud. With such disturbances there usually is impairment in abstract thinking and more or less general mental damage.

    1. *Physiological background:* The exact anatomical lesions producing this type of aphasia are subject to debate by all authorities known to us. Wernicke decided causative lesions must be in the region of the insula Reili and that injury to association fibers connecting motor and speech areas was always present. Goldstein insisted there must also be dysfunction of cortical apparatus and cited various cases from Bischoff, Bleuler, Pick, and von Monakov to substantiate his position.

        Goldstein admitted the important bearing of the insula Reili on central motor aphasia but included the adjacent areas of the temporal and parietal lobes in the central speech areas, calling special attention to the cases described by Stengel and by Liepmann and Pappenheim, in which the lesion had not affected the insula Reili. Stengel's case involved damage to the posterior two-thirds of the second temporal convolution extending into the gyrus angularis and the lower part of the first temporal convolution.

Further, Goldstein considered involvement of the temporal lobes as most important in any occurrence of central aphasia. He called particular attention to the extensive convolutions and various subcortical fiber systems entering the insula Reili, suggesting the tractus longitudinalis inferior must play a specific part in repetition since it connects those sections of the temporal and frontal lobes considered of vital importance for language.

2. *Symptoms:*

   a. Those usually manifested are similar to symptoms found in pure motor (peripheral) aphasia. There is impaired ability in word-finding, singing, and in using spontaneous speech. Spontaneous speech may be totally absent. In peripheral motor aphasia there is no disturbance in the realm of inner language but the central motor aphasic is markedly impaired, exhibiting general mental damage and inability to think abstractly along with more or less difficulty in understanding.

   b. Patient shows lack of ability to speak on command.

   c. Because of impaired abstract attitude, patient's speech may exhibit motor defects. However, motor disturbances of the speech automatisms (sounds, words, phrases, sentences) are not so pronounced as in pure motor aphasia. Patient may be able to utter many words correctly.

   d. Patient seems unable to initiate a word or number series but, given the first item of the series, will frequently produce the complete series without motoric defect and with normal speech rhythm.

e. Patient appears to think concretely and may even utter concrete language but cannot express abstract ideas.

f. He can use conversational speech so long as he can think in concrete terms.

g. Patient tends to speak very little.

h. He can usually repeat words in the concrete realm. However, he flounders when attempting voluntarily to repeat an abstract word.

i. Patient's speech may evidence agrammatism and the use of telegram style (see Agrammatism, page 26). It is difficult for him to say "small" words, particularly when isolated or in the context of abstract material.

j. Patient may exert efforts to speak voluntarily but perseverance is of no avail in speech improvement.

k. He has difficulty in reading aloud, although that may be easier than for him to speak.

    1^a. Usually concrete words are more easily read than are abstract ones.

    2^a. Small words appearing in abstract phrases or sentences may be omitted when he reads.

    3^a. Patient may comprehend partially or completely what he reads aloud.

    4^a. Usually material read silently is more readily understood than material he reads aloud.

l. Patient cannot write "small" words in isolation or when they appear in abstract matter although he may produce them in connection with concrete material.

m. Writing is particularly disturbed when there is difficulty in combining letters into words. He may or may not be able to intonate. Letters may be formed correctly but omitted in words or changed in their proper order. The disturbance in writing usually mirrors the speech defect.

n. Some patients exhibit amnesic aphasia and auditory agnosia along with the central aphasia.

3. *Amnesic Aphasia*

I. *Definition:* A disruption of language pattern formulations manifested by patient's inability to find suitable names to use for concrete objects (e.g., table, chair) when trying to explain a problem or analyze a situation—that is, when he is attempting to assume a conceptual viewpoint or employ an abstract attitude. (See pages 15–17 and 82–86.) His concern is not the world about him, but himself. He thinks in terms of *me*. Amnesic aphasia pertains to the forgetting of names and is sometimes termed *nominal aphasia*.

II. *Physiological Background:* It may appear in lesions of temporal, parietal, and frontal lobes. Amnesic aphasias resulting solely from frontal lesions are rare and Nielsen noted that if frontal lesions do produce amnesic aphasia, they must be due to "interruption of associations between the temporal and frontal areas."[30] Goldstein noticed that the clearest development of this symptom complex (amnesic aphasia) occurred when the lesion was located in the temporoparietal region, which meant that speech areas were affected too. He felt a lesion of Broca's speech area alone is never followed by amnesic aphasia defect in word-finding. [31]

[30] *Ibid.*, p. 72.
[31] Goldstein, Kurt: *Language and Language Disturbances,* Grune & Stratton, Inc., New York, 1948, p. 290.

III. *Symptoms:*

   A. Patient's speech is practically void of concrete words. Nouns, adjectives, adverbs, and auxiliary verbs are often missing. This difficulty in finding concrete words tends to make an amnesic aphasic use paraphrases and circumlocutions.

   B. Patient has difficulty in recalling familiar names such as those of his wife, the city in which he lives, and the street in front of his home. He may remember a name at one moment but cannot recall it a few moments later. He may produce intelligible speech at one time, while a little later his speech may become all but impossible because there are so many names he has forgotten.

   C. Patient frequently becomes emotionally upset over the inability to recall names.

   D. There usually is impairment in ability to tell the size and color of an object. Producing such a description as chartreuse green, copper brown, lemon yellow, etc., is impossible for the amnesic. Given a list of concrete nouns, the patient rejects incorrect words for concrete objects but immediately recognizes the correct word when it is spoken. He tends toward voluble speaking.

   E. Patient is totally unable to assume a conceptual viewpoint. His abstract attitude is impaired.

   F. Propositional speech is an impossibility.

   G. There may be disturbance in the instrumentalities of speech although the problem is not motoric as in central motor aphasia. Damage to the instrumentalities (the sounds, words, phrases, sentences, emotional utterances, series of words, and some forms of naming) resembles somewhat the disturbance a normal person displays when pronouncing a foreign word. Patient may try to pronounce a word although it may have no meaning to him. The amnesic aphasic tends to pronounce words as though trying to pronounce a foreign word that has no meaning to him. He may produce the sounds of the word correctly but will not comprehend the word.

H. So far as we know, motor speech difficulties never appear in pure amnesia.

I. When patient has difficulty in recalling a certain word and it is said for him, he can repeat that word easily. He recognizes the correct word when it is given to him.

J. Being given the initial or key sound of a word does not help the true amnesic aphasic.

K. When requested to count or recite the alphabet or name the days of the weeks, etc., he has difficulty in starting. However, if the first or second member of the series is given, he is likely to proceed. He may forget how a word "looks" or sounds; or be unable to remember how the speech musculature must be used in producing the word.

L. He finds it difficult to stop at a certain point in a series when requested. When interrupted within a series, it is almost impossible for him to proceed with that series.

M. Paraphasia occasionally is evidenced. (See Paraphasia, pages 24–28.)

N. Alexia is sometimes revealed. (See discussion of alexia, page 23.)

O. Paragraphia is evidenced at times. (See Paragraphia, page 28.)

   1. Patient actually thinks concretely and may write concrete words more easily than abstract words, but small words in isolation like *in*, *the*, *and*, etc., are exceedingly difficult. They may have no meaning to him.

   2. Patient may be unable to write spontaneously but may copy or write from dictation with comparative accuracy. This inability to write spontaneously is frequently termed *amnesic agraphia* or *paragraphia*.

3. Patient may substitute words when writing from dictation. However, when patient Tom was asked to write (and say), "I eat my turkey," he wrote, "I eat the me turkey." As he wrote the letters *t-h-e*, he said *eat*; when he wrote *m-e*, he said *my*.

P. Patient frequently tends to speak a great deal.

CHAPTER V

APPRAISAL OF THE PATIENT'S CAPACITIES

ACCURATE APPRAISAL OF A PATIENT'S SPEECH AND LANGUAGE capacities is a primary and vital requirement in dealing with the aphasic. In fact, speech and language observations (together with neurological and clinical findings) are the only correct basis for determining diagnosis and treatment.

The therapist's goal when dealing with aphasics—or any patients with personality problems—always ought to be greater understanding of total personal functioning. One can start with what the patient offers or manifests as a complaint and then make inquiries upon which to elaborate, formulate, and treat. At the same time, all obtainable case history data from every legitimate source should be weighed and correlated with signs presented by the patient. Factual material from parents or relatives should be obtained from each one separately so that discrepancies may be revealed. These can be helpful in formulating a program for therapy.

Natal and developmental material should be sought which will explain the patient's social adaptations. What were his interests and dislikes while a student in grade or high school or college? What of his present interests and habits, especially eating, sleeping, playing, working, etc.? Watch patient closely to observe his appearance, behavior, and activities during the first interview, the changing moods, etc. Check the orientation and rapport. Does he appear open, frank, and confiding, or guarded and hostile? Note especially his intellectual resources and the ability to retain or recall.

If the therapist believes the problem is aphasia, the question should be asked: Is it organic or functional in origin or a combination of these? Our clinical experience indicates that aphasic cases of primary organic involvement always present some functional (i.e., psychological) problems as well. Every organic aphasic seems to exhibit both a psychological and structural involvement.

A. Differential Diagnosis

In order to make a thorough diagnosis, speech and language symptoms must be differentiated and studied in all of their complex forms. One of the first major problems is to determine whether or not the patient has an aphasia. Not infrequently a patient has been diagnosed as such when actually there *was* no aphasia! Instead, he had one or more of the following conditions:

1. Defective hearing or vision resulting from pathological involvement of the organs.
2. Hysterical aphonia.
3. Severe dysarthria (caused by a lesion of the central nervous system, from which or by which the organs of articulation are controlled).
4. Mental retardation.
5. Neurotic and psychotic states.

While some or all of these can and frequently do appear in *conjunction* with aphasia, *they* are not, by definition, aphasia! The literature indicates that any one of the five listed disorders may appear without aphasia.

When making diagnostic tests to determine the presence of aphasia, the examiner must seek to discover any defective functions. Are these visual or auditory? Does the patient have difficulty in the use of objects or the use of his speech musculature? Can he use and comprehend language and if so, to what extent? What does the examiner consider to be the patient's greatest losses? In what field does the *patient* feel he has the greatest losses? (His observations may differ markedly from the examiner's beliefs.) Observation of the defective functions may prove most helpful in locating intracranial pathologies. However, the disturbing lesion or neoplasm may be some distance away from the area affected, since edema and pressure rapidly encroach upon various adjacent areas of the brain.

Next, consider the way in which the aphasic's performance capacities (his responses) indicate residual ability. That is, what are the *undamaged* areas? Such information of the patient's needs is essential in planning the therapy program. (See Chapters VII and VIII.)

It is necessary to approach the aphasic patient in one of two ways or in both, depending on the nature and severity of the difficulty:

1. Concentrate upon the function in which the patient feels he has the greatest loss.
2. Exploit the residual capacities of the patient and use them as a means of approaching the integrative functions.

B. Case Study

The initial step in making any speech and language appraisal of a brain-injured individual is the obtaining of a thorough case history. The first contact with the patient should never involve securing detailed information from him. Obtain all possible case history data from the referring physician and the family prior to the first interview with the patient. The most helpful information should cover the following:

1. Name, address, and telephone number of the patient.

Name, address, and telephone number of nearest relative and/or legal guardian.

2. Name by which the patient likes to be called. Names of
his immediate family; how the patient addresses each
member (nicknames, etc.).
3. Where and when patient was born.
4. Where he spent his childhood.
5. His childhood home life.
6. Early schooling.
7. Early language background.
8. Premorbid handedness of patient. Familial tendencies
of handedness.
9. Present home or hospital environment. Names of those
now taking care of him.
10. Family attitude toward patient.
11. His premorbid intellectual capacities. Was an I.Q.
taken before the onset? If so, what was the score? The
Wepman[1] studies indicate there is some predictive
value in pretraumatic intellectual scores.
12. High school or college training.
13. His premorbid profession or occupation. A bookkeep-
er's loss of ability to add a column of figures is a far
greater ego blow than the same loss would be to a
housewife.
14. His premorbid personality characteristics.
15. Any present personality deviations. How does patient
express his needs and drives? Though his basic personality does not change after trauma, there may be a
shift in the methods and ways of revealing inner
desires and needs.
16. Patient's premorbid hobbies. Does he enjoy doing anything now? Television? Radio? Newspapers? Maga-
zines?

[1] Wepman, J. M.: *Recovery from Aphasia.* The Ronald Press Co., New York,
1951, p. 75.

17. Names, addresses, and telephone numbers of attending physicians. It is important to get the names of doctors from whom medical reports may be obtained.
18. Previous medical and surgical history. Reports of ophthalmological and audiometer tests, encephalograms, etc.
19. Description of patient's present complaints.

It is highly desirable to have a medical report—oral or written—from attending physicians because the medical picture prior to the first consultation equips the aphasia therapist to appraise the patient's speech and language capacities more effectively.

We have found the case study methods created by Henry Head and set forth in his book, *Aphasia and Kindred Disorders of Speech*, Volume I, pages 145–65 (The Macmillan Company, New York, 1926) and the methods used by Adolf Meyer, late dean emeritus of Henry Phipps School of Psychiatry at Johns Hopkins University, helpful in appraising the aphasic.

Meyer devised his examination techniques primarily for psychiatric patients but they are highly appropriate and adaptable for clinical observations of an aphasic's speech and language capacities. We concur with Meyer's findings that the aphasic's problems can be attacked only through a full analysis of his responses. For a detailed outline of all the examination steps used by Dr. Meyer, refer to the second edition of Muncie's *Psychobiology and Psychiatry*, pages 151–92 and 381–89 (C. W. Mosby Co., St. Louis, 1948).

C. TESTING

1. *Early Stages of Therapy*

After obtaining all available preliminary case history information, the next step is general testing of the patient's capacities. At this first session, only a general appraisal should be made. Tests are often frustrating and fatiguing to an aphasic and may even cause catastrophic reactions. Therefore, we find it better not to attempt to do a great deal of testing at this first consultation. Our observation is that it is better to space testing sessions at various intervals over a four- to six-week period.

Let the first consultation be brief—seldom or never over 45 minutes. The major aim at this initial session is to determine whether or not therapy is indicated. If treatment is recommended, then we discuss with the patient in general terms what can be done to help him express himself.

As in all therapy sessions, it is important to make this first contact a happy experience (not only to give the patient reassurance that something definite can be done to make his life meaningful) but to create a feeling that he is wanted and necessary to the world. Build all possible rapport with him. *Do* something to make him feel he is actually starting toward a goal. (See Chapter VII, "Initial Therapeutic Considerations."

When giving tests to an aphasic, always conduct the examination (and later therapy) in comfortable surroundings with easy chairs and pleasing draperies. Only the patient and therapist should be in the room, for any type of extraneous stimulus is most distracting to the aphasic. Soft carpeting and sound-proofing are advantageous. Because of the aphasic's low frustration tolerance and rapid fatigability, he is easily disturbed by little things. Sometimes even a change of furniture in an office or room will disturb him greatly.

Always assume a permissive attitude when giving tests. Encourage the patient and give him plenty of time to relax while testing. Keep in mind his problem of fatigability.

During all testing, record everything he says. As soon as directions for a test are given, remain silent while the individual is trying to respond. If any remark or question is interposed, record both what you say and the patient's reply. Keep asking yourself: "How can this problem be attacked?" "What avenues of entry are open to this person's consciousness?" Only by arousing his interest can the therapist induce the patient to respond in the early stages of therapy.

Study the patient in this testing situation to learn his needs. Appraise all symptoms or reactions with reference to the present situation. Even though he fails to complete a given task in a performance test, do not decide that he lacks the ability to do it. He may fail through fear or err from feelings of apprehension and anxiety. Hence you must study his reactions in the light of the total behavior situation.

Record the exact responses. What did he say and how did he say it? What did he do? Carefully observe all facial and bodily expressions of fear, anxiety, or emotional upset. Make notes of those which were apparent. All these factors are important in getting a true picture of your aphasic patient.

Speech and language tests are subject to certain provisos. Avoid thinking in terms of plus or minus; of whether a performance is right or wrong. The motive for giving these tests is not to see what score the patient can make. No score should ever be assigned to an aphasic because no two aphasics can ever be compared. A peculiarity of an aphasic's problem is that he may perform adequately in the more advanced levels of a certain test but fail utterly in the lower levels of that same test. *Qualitative* results are the important aspects to be studied, not his *quantitative* results.

It is undesirable to make all of these tests at the first session. Not more than two or three of them should be given; certainly not more than eight or ten. The number of tests used will depend *entirely* upon the individual patient—the severity of his problem, his willingness and eagerness for help, and how soon he shows any signs of restlessness or fatigue.

If or when the patient fails in any one of the tests, be sure to modify the task in such a way that he can accomplish it. When he shows he is tired, give him a task you feel he can do successfully, then terminate the session and arrange for another one at a later date. As in all future therapy sessions, it is very important to end this first consultation on a successful note, thus vitally motivating future therapeutic meetings with this patient.

In all testing of an aphasic, keep a record of the speech with which the patient performs each test. The ease, rapidity, and skill with which any task is carried out is significant when appraising the patient's abilities. Do not record the test time obtrusively and *never mention* the *time* element to the patient. If he does a test rapidly and well, praise him enthusiastically. You will note that usually the tasks that are performed skillfully and with ease are those requiring the shortest length of time between question (stimulus) and response.

During the first interview, your primary goal is to make a general appraisal of the patient to determine if he can hear and comprehend spoken language. Does he seem in a stupor or is he aware of the world about him? When entering the room, greet the patient with "How are you today, ———? As your physician has told you, I am ———, a specialist in speech problems. I'm here to help you." If not in a stupor and if he actually wants help, these introductory remarks will usually bring forth a friendly response. Then continue, "I am going to ask you a few very simple questions."

TEST ONE: Directions: "Do you have an eye? . . . Point to your eye. . . . Do you have an ear? . . . Point to your ear. . . . A nose? . . . Point to your nose. . . . A mouth? . . . Point to your mouth. . . . An arm? . . . Point to your arm. . . . A hand? . . . Point to your hand. . . . Hair? . . . Point to your hair," etc. By asking questions for each body part, the examiner can better test the patient's ability to understand. Test One will determine whether the patient has a problem in recognizing and understanding.

1. If there is difficulty in recognizing an object he sees, the

problem may be *visual agnosia* (or a hysterical amblyopia, a unilateral or bilateral homonymous hemianopia,
or a defect in visual fields).

2. If there is difficulty in recognizing body parts, the problem is called *body agnosia*, *topagnosia*, or *autotopagnosia*. If the patient cannot designate certain fingers on
   command, the disturbance is *finger agnosia*.

3. If there is difficulty in understanding what is said to
   him, there may be one or several problems to be solved.
   The examination must discover what the patient has
   difficulty in understanding, because:

   a. If he cannot hear, the problem may result from
      pathology of the auricular mechanism or it may
      be a cortical deafness arising from bilateral de-
      struction of the transverse temporal gyrus.

   b. If he cannot associate a perceived sound with its
      meaning, *auditory agnosia* is probable.

   c. There may be deficiency in mentality or mental
      impairment. If so, the cause must be ascertained.

   d. There may be disturbance in abstract attitude (i.e.,
      impairment in inner speech). This disturbance
      may be due to damage in the thinking instru-
      mentalities or independent of them. (See pages
      82–86.)

During this test, the patient may understand what you ask
but lack the ability to carry out instructions. In that case, the
problem may be *apraxia*. (See also Head's Hand, Ear, and
Eye Test in *Aphasia and Kindred Disorders of Speech*, Volume I, pages 157–60.)

Only by careful analysis of all presenting signs and by
future thorough testing can the examiner determine the actual field or fields of defect and decide whether it involves
one or several; whether a defect in one area causes defect in
another area or whether the observed disorder is a secondary
result of some other disturbance. As an illustration of the

latter: a difficulty in word-finding may develop from actual mental impairment, or the patient's mentation may be disturbed by his problem of finding words to express himself.

TEST TWO: If patient evidenced ability to understand in Test One, give in sequence directions such as: "Point to your left eye. . . . Point to your right ear, . . . your left arm, . . . your left ear," etc. If there is difficulty in determining spacial relationships between any part of his body and other objects or if he confuses the right and left sides of the body, his problem is *agnosia for space.*

TEST THREE: After patient has successfully performed Test One, print each command on a sheet of paper (e.g., *Point to your ear*), and proceed as in Test One. If he succeeded in the first test but fails this one, the problem is *visual verbal agnosia.*

TEST FOUR: Should patient understand audible speech in Test One, ask him to count the fingers on your hand (or on his). If there is difficulty in starting the series—that is, in saying number one—the problem may be one of naming or word-finding or difficulty in forming speech sounds or impairment of abstract attitude.

TEST FIVE: Test patient's ability to recognize objects in the room. Give such directions as "Point to the chair. . . . Point to the desk. . . . Point to the lamp, . . . to the bed (or couch), . . . to the mirror, . . . to the door," etc. If these directions are heeded, most likely there is no difficulty in the realm of words (i.e., there is no *auditory verbal agnosia*).

TEST SIX: Test patient's ability to name objects in the room as you point to them. Point to the pen and ask, "What is this?"; point to the knife and query, "What is this?"; to the lamp, etc. Try him with eight or ten objects. If he fails to name an object, do not at once repeat the question but ask it again during this test. Some are able to name an object at one moment but fail at another time and it is most important to make a series of observations before deciding upon your diagnosis. If patient fails Test Six, the problem may be one or more of the following:

1. Impairment of abstract attitude.
2. Amnesic aphasia evidenced by patient's inability to respond with the correct word. Even though he responds, he may use circumlocutions. For instance, in the effort to say *knife*, an amnesic aphasic might say, "Something you cut with." If he wished to say *pen* but could not recall that word, he might say, "Something you write with."
3. Visual agnosia. Inability to recognize an object seen. (See Test One, page 68.)
4. Geometric-optic agnosia. Inability to recognize an object seen although the peripheral visual mechanism may be intact. The major difficulty is in recognizing form which may create a disturbance in reading (alexia) or writing (agraphia).
5. Auditory agnosia. Inability to recognize spoken language.
6. Echolalia. Patient may respond to your question, "What is this?" by saying, "What is this?"
7. Paraphasia. Patient may explain an object rather than name it. In explanations or conversations he may omit words. Such telegram language is called *paraphasia*. If grammar is ignored, the particular problem is acataphasia or agrammatism. (See pages 26–27.)
8. Apraxia of the speech muscles.
9. Transcortical sensory aphasia or transcortical motor aphasia.
10. Central motor aphasia.

11. Combined expressive-receptive aphasia.
12. Global aphasia. If patient lacks all speech, he is said to be a global aphasic, having lost completely the ability to communicate. His writing ability should then be tested. (See Test Twenty-two on page 79.) If he writes meaningful sentences, inner speech is not disturbed. In addition, test the global aphasic's ability to sing. He may be able to sing at least one word although unable to say anything. (See Test Seventeen on page 77.)

There is always the possibility that patient is a polyglot, so test him for other languages. Find out from the family if he spoke more than one language premorbidly. If so, ask him to say a specific word in as many languages as he can. Unable to produce it in one language, he may do so in another language. This has occurred in our practice.

TEST SEVEN: If patient succeeds in Test Three, check his ability to recognize spoken numbers. Place ten pencils or matches or sticks in front of patient and say, "Give me *two* pencils, . . . *one* pencil, . . . *five* pencils, . . . *three* pencils, . . . *eight* pencils," etc. Failure in this test indicates auditory agnosia in the realm of numbers—*auditory number agnosia.*

TEST EIGHT: Test patient's orientation to time. Direct him to show on a model clock the position of the hands at six o'clock, . . . three o'clock, . . . eight o'clock, . . . etc. If he reveals difficulty in this, there may be *agnosia for time* or the problem may be *auditory agnosia.* Before ruling out auditory agnosia, print the hours at which the clock is to be set (e.g., four:ten; six:thirty; eight:fifteen; etc.). If unable to solve this problem, there may be *visual verbal agnosia.* Write the hours numerically (e.g., 4:10; 6:30; 8:15) and test him. If he succeeds, there may be difficulty in word-naming. Numbers as such may be concrete objects to him, thus permitting recognition of them. See the Clock Test in *Aphasia and Kindred Disorders of Speech* by Henry Head, Volume I, page 157.)

TEST NINE:

1. Place five vividly contrasting colored crayons (we use red, blue, green, yellow, orange) in a row on a table at left front of the patient. Lay five identically colored crayons on the same table but at right front of the patient, covering these with a sheet of paper. Select one of the "hidden" crayons and ask patient to give you a crayon "just like it" from the exposed group at his left. Patients unable to identify many colors are thought to be color blind, but they actually may succeed on this test, which indicates they are not color blind. Inability to match colors in this test shows the problem is probably one of *visual color agnosia.*

2. Should patient match the colors, ask him to point to pencils of various colors on the table (e.g., point to a red or a green or a yellow pencil). If he has difficulty, the problem is *visual color agnosia.*

3. After success on parts 1 and 2, tell him to *name* the color of each pencil and the color of various objects in the room. Failure to name these may be due to *nominal aphasia* or to *apraxia.* (See pages 57 and 37.)

TEST TEN:

1. Should patient be unable to employ spontaneous speech in Test Nine, direct him to: "Repeat after me the word *pen,* . . . *ink,* . . . *lamp,* . . . *desk*," etc. Repeating a requested word evidences that the minor hemisphere played a part in premorbid speech processes and is now operating in the postmorbid speech picture. (See pages 5–6.) Auditory verbal agnosia is ruled out because he understood and heeded your spoken directions.

2. Hand the patient a sheet on which is printed the state-

ment "Point to the large box" along with two pictured boxes (as shown).

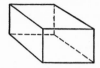

Tell him to read aloud and remember what he read. Now ask him to follow the instruction he just read.

a. If patient comprehends what he has read but cannot select the large-sized box, the problem is *visual size agnosia.*

b. If he read the sentence aloud accurately but did not comprehend it, *transcortical sensory aphasia* is present.

c. Test further for transcortical aphasia by directing him as follows: "Repeat this sentence after me. 'Point to the star.' " (The three objects shown can be made of cardboard.)

If the patient repeats accurately but does not heed the direction, his problem is either *transcortical sensory aphasia* or *transcortical motor aphasia.* Some patients repeating material over and over begin to catch its meaning. Such is the case in *transcortical sensory aphasia.* If unable to repeat the sentence, the problem may be *central motor aphasia.* A central motor aphasic usually can repeat a concrete word but not an abstract one.

d. If he cannot read the sentences, the problem may be *visual agnosia.* (See Tests Eight, Nine, and

Ten.) If he reads but doesn't understand the sentences, his difficulty is aphasic. (See point *a* above.)

e. When patient reverses sounds or syllables within a word or reverses phrases, his difficulty is *paraphasia.*

f. The patient who drools or reads laboriously with abrupt increases or decreases in volume and sudden interruptions in articulation has *dysarthria.* For an additional test of dysarthria, ask patient to repeat after you, *Massachusetts* and *Methodist Episcopal Church.* Again, if he speaks with stress and strain and with sudden breaks in voice production, or there are sounds substituted or omitted along with sudden changes in volume or a "whiny" voice, the problem is *dysarthria.*

TEST ELEVEN: Should the previous tests produce unintelligible jargon, write or print in colored pencil on a large sheet of paper the following words:

boy	girl
cat	bear
mother	tiger
lion	mother
father	rabbit

Direct patient to: "Pick out the animals, . . . the people . . . ." Should he select the correct words, there is no severe semantic problem and he has more or less residual reading ability.

TEST TWELVE: Count aloud from 1 to 100. Then count by 5's to 100. Inability to count aloud in series indicates apraxia of the speech musculature. Should the patient be unable to write numbers in series, there may be apraxia of the hand muscles (*apractic agraphia*) or *isolated agraphia.* When he has difficulty in starting a number series but counts successfully after being given the first member of the series, there may be apraxia of the speech muscles. However, there may be present pure motor aphasia or central motor aphasia. The transcortical motor aphasic is helped when given the first number of a series but cannot proceed with the series even though he tries diligently to do so. As a further check, ask him to write the symbols 1 to 100. If he succeeds, have him write these symbols: *four*, *6*, *nine*, *8*, *17*. Give the directions: "Read these." Avoid all use of the word *number* when giving these directions. If he fails, *visual number agnosia* is evidenced.

TEST THIRTEEN: Following success in Test Twelve, instruct him to: "Write the words: *four, two, eight*." If he fails, the difficulty may be due to *auditory agnosia*, *agraphia*, or *apraxia*. (See Tests One to Six.)

TEST FOURTEEN: Write out on a sheet of paper or a blackboard some simple arithmetic problems suitable to the patient's premorbid education and experience in calculation. For instance, if he had only an elementary schooling, use problems such as:

$$
\begin{array}{ccccccc}
234 & 143 & 124 & 247 & 387 & 195 & 187 \\
\times\ 26 & +324 & +168 & +179 & -146 & -136 & -\ 98 \\
\end{array}
$$

$$36 - 4 = ? \quad 3\overline{)489}$$
$$30 - 3 = ? \quad 9 \times 12 =$$

This test helps to determine the general degree of loss in the realm of calculation. If patient fails in it, the problem involves *calculation apraxia*. (See pages 41–42.)

TEST FIFTEEN: With a musician patient, ask him to select on a musical staff specific notes as you name them. If instructions are understood but not heeded, the problem involves *visual music agnosia*.

TEST SIXTEEN: Test patient's ability to recognize and distinguish noises. Tell him to: "Point out the object which is 'making the sound.'" Use a whistle or maid's bell; close a drawer or a door. If he understands directions but fails the test, his problem is *auditory agnosia*.

TEST SEVENTEEN: Hum "America." Patient may not be able to tell you the song is "America" but actions may show he recognized it. If there is no recognition, the problem is auditory in the musical realm—that is *auditory music agnosia* or *amusia*. Amusia may also be evidenced by testing his ability to recognize instruments being played, and his capacity to discern whether music is being played slowly or fast. Some patients respond: "I know the name of that song but just can't say it." This circumlocution is typical of an amnesic aphasic. It is also found often in perfectly normal people, including your authors.

After humming "America," ask: "What was I doing?" If patient cannot tell you were humming, his difficulty could involve:

1. An agnosia which may be either visual or auditory or kinesthetic, or all of these.
2. An apraxia.
3. Nominal aphasia.

TEST EIGHTEEN: Instruct patient as follows: "Close your eyes and as I place an object in your hand, please tell me if it is a watch, pencil, fork, spoon, or penny." If unable to name the object but he seems to understand oral directions, say: "Close your eyes. There are five objects on the desk in front of you: a watch, pencil, fork, spoon, and a penny. I shall ask you for one of them. Please feel these objects and hand me the one I ask for. [Pause.] Fork. . . . Penny. . . . Spoon. . . ." etc. If the directions are understood but he can't select the objects through feel or touch, the problem may be *tactile agnosia* or it may be anomia (difficulty in word-finding) or apraxia.

TEST NINETEEN: Ask patient to write his name. If unable to write at all, he has *agraphia*. If there is difficulty in writing, print the word in large letters on a sheet of paper or on a blackboard and ask that he copy it. Then have him copy simple figures such as $\bigcirc$, $+$, $\triangle$, $\square$, $\perp$; then more complicated ones like $\triangle$, $\sqsubset$, $\underset{+}{\sqcup}$, $\triangle$. If unable to copy accurately, the problem may be *visual agnosia* or it may be *apraxia*.

TEST TWENTY: If patient tries in Test Nineteen to write with the wrong end of the pencil or cannot use one, ask him to perform manual acts such as lighting a cigarette, cutting with scissors, etc. If he is unable to perform these acts or seems unfamiliar with the use of the objects or uses them absent-mindedly (inadvertently puts lighted end of cigarette in mouth), the difficulty is *apraxia of the hand muscles*.

TEST TWENTY-ONE: Seat patient directly in front of you and tell him to: "Do everything I do." Protrude tongue; smack lips; put tongue on upper lip; put tongue at right of lip; etc. If he cannot perform these acts when sitting in front of the therapist, seat patient before a mirror and sit beside him. Proceed with task as above. If he still cannot mimic the various movements of your speech musculature, *apraxia of the speech muscles* is evidenced. (It is more difficult for the aphasic patient to mimic acts when sitting opposite therapist than when both he and therapist are looking in the mirror.) Head points out that the majority of aphasics have little difficulty in mimicking movements reflected in a mirror, but this has not been the observation of the authors in testing aphasics, particularly those handicapped in the expressive realm. In fact, apraxia of speech muscles is frequently evidenced by aphasics being utterly unable to mimic movements reflected in the mirror.

TEST TWENTY-TWO: When patient fails to name objects in Test Five (page 70), direct him to: "Write the name of the object" (knife, lamp, etc.). If he writes the noun, it indicates he "knows" but cannot reproduce the word orally. The problem probably is *expressive aphasia*—either pure motor or apraxia. (See pages 37–52.) If unable to write the word, his difficulty may be:

1. Paragraphia. (See page 28.)
2. Apraxia. (See page 37.)
3. Nominal aphasia. (See pages 57–60.)
4. Visual agnosia. (See pages 22–30.)

Patient may write his own name but fail if asked to write the names of parents, sons, daughters, etc.

TEST TWENTY-THREE: If patient can use a pencil, ask him to draw a diagram of the hospital room or consulting room. If he fails, the problem may be *construction apraxia.*

TEST TWENTY-FOUR: When unable to grasp a pencil because of apraxia, give patient a set of cards with large letters or some blocks with raised letters on them and proceed with Tests Nineteen to Twenty-two. If he can spell with the large letters or blocks but cannot write, *construction apraxia* is ruled out.

TEST TWENTY-FIVE: If patient cannot use a paralyzed hand, usually the right (see pages 5–6), suggest that he use the "other" hand to write his name. If he holds the pencil and recognizes its use but can't write his name correctly, there may be one or several reasons:

1. Damage to the second frontal convolution may have produced a motor agraphia, which could be a primary defect unconnected with any difficulty he may have in expressive aphasia.
2. Visualization disturbances may be arising from eye pathology or a visual agnosia.

3. Inability to speak (pure word mutism) which may not be the cause per se of the agraphia. If premorbidly patient "said" or "whispered" a word as he wrote it, the postmorbid writing ability will certainly be influenced by this earlier habit pattern. An expressive aphasia (mutism) patient who did not premorbidly accompany his writing with whispers or spoken words would not necessarily have an agraphia.

4. Impairment of abstract attitude manifested by defective inner speech (cortical sensory aphasia) would also disturb his writing ability. Should he write concrete words more easily, it is because they do not require employment of abstract attitude.

5. The difficulty may be *literal paragraphia* or *agrammatic paragraphia*, revealed by the patient misspelling his name when writing it. This paragraphia results from the agrammatic difficulty. (See pages 28–29.)

6. If the name is written "phonetically" (as it actually sounds), his problem is *written paraphasia*.

7. A polyglot patient may be able to write his name in one language but not in another. With such a patient, test him on *all* his languages.

8. When written or printed letters appear distorted or are written backwards, mirror writing may be indicated. (See pages 111–12.)

9. If patient cannot write his name, write it in large letters and ask him to copy it. Does he copy the script precisely or use his own style of handwriting? If he forms the letters in the wrong direction, the problem may be *geometric-optic agnosia*. (See Test Three.)

10. If patient writes his own name legibly, have him write the name of the city in which he lives. If unable to recall that name, he has *amnesic aphasia*. If unable to write it, the problem is *amnesic aphasic agraphia*.

11. After patient copies his name in script, have him copy

it from print. If he succeeds, print a word (e.g., *boy*) and tell him to write it in his own handwriting. A patient who can copy the figures in Test Nineteen may fail in this test, which shows he is not copying the symbol (letter) but is reading the letter and then trying to write it. In such case, the problem would be in the realm of writing what has been read—not actually copying the symbol.

12. Should patient write his name or the word *boy* spontaneously, with accuracy, tell him to write *girl*. If he fails, the problem may be *auditory agnosia*. (See Test One.) He may write the word *girl* but not know *what* he has written because the word may have no meaning to him. Check carefully on this by showing him pictures of a boy, a girl, and two other objects (e.g., chair, table). Have him point out the object whose name he has written. If he cannot select the correct objects, his problem is in the realm of *alexia*.

TEST TWENTY-SIX: If patient seemed to have poor vision or difficulty in visual agnosia in Test Twenty-five, ask him to write with the eyes closed.

TEST TWENTY-SEVEN: Show a picture and ask patient to tell what is happening in the picture. This is a more complicated test comprising various tasks appraised in the above tests. Difficulties which may be evidenced are:
1. Impairment of ability to handle abstract ideas.
2. Word-finding.
3. Paraphasia.
4. Visual agnosia.
5. Circumlocutions.

TEST TWENTY-EIGHT: Tell patient to read silently a human interest story in the magazine or newspaper. When he has finished reading, have him give the idea of the story. If he had difficulty in reading silently, the problem may be *alexia*. Tell him to read another human interest story aloud. If he can do this but does not comprehend the material, his problem may be *transcortical sensory aphasia*. If concrete words seem easier for the patient to read than the abstract ones, the difficulty may be *central motor aphasia*. Also, central motor aphasia is evidenced if patient omits small words when they appear in abstract phrases and if silent reading seems to be understood more readily than oral reading.

A major consideration in these general appraisal tests is the degree of normality of the patient's mental functioning. Aphasia problems often precipitate various disturbances in intelligence, and impaired intellectual capacities can create difficulties. Brain injury may cause defective intelligence with a contingent aphasia, or brain damage may cause aphasia with a consequently impaired intelligence. Again, aphasia and defective intelligence may occur as entirely separate syndromes. In such cases, the area of mental damage is apart from the aphasia damage. This actually occurs in auditory aphasia. The patient may be deficient in comprehension for two reasons: he may have difficulty in understanding what he actually hears; in addition, he may have impaired intelligence. Either problem may be entirely separate from the other.

Although aphasia involves changes in mental functioning, it does not necessarily include general intellectual defect. The essential disorder is loss in the "know-how" of speech and language on the part of the aphasic.

When making this preliminary appraisal of the aphasic, certain major factors should be considered. Is the patient failing because of defective intelligence or erring because of actual deficiency in a specific performance? Is there a disturbance of speech automatisms—sounds, words, sentences, word series, and/or emotional utterances? Is there a disturbance in reading? in writing? in spelling? Is he failing because of an actual fear of not succeeding? Or is his problem an inability to think abstractly, that is, can he think only in concrete terms?

Normal conversational speech includes both concrete and abstract terms. The meaning of a word is determined not only by its background but its use in the context. For example, in a painting which depicts a ship on a calm sea at sunset, the ship is normally the most noticeable object. An observer may be aware that the object is a ship, but the painting has little meaning until he considers the implications of the background—and what is *behind* the ship. Considered in relation to the calm sea and the multicolored sky, it takes on real meaning. Against the background of a turbulent sea and an angry-looking sky, the significance of the painted ship would be quite different. So with a word, its meaning to a listener is a combination of the attitudes and tone of voice of the speaker, plus what its background and context reveals. This ability to establish relationships between words and their context or between a figure and the background in a picture is a simple experience for the normal individual but a difficult one for a brain-injured person. When the cortex has been damaged, the ability to differentiate between a painted figure and its background may be so markedly disturbed that the patient confuses the two. He may say one thing and actually mean the opposite. When patient Frances wishes to say *Mother*, she utters *home*; when she means *yes*, she often comes forth with *no*. If patient Herbert wants to count from one to ten, he frequently starts the alphabetical series *a, b, c, d*, etc. These are typical symptoms of the brain-injured.

Jackson believed that many aphasics had not confused or lost the meaning of a word but were unable to use a specific word for a particular purpose. For example, when the normal person says "car" in reference to his own automobile, he visualizes a specific car. But when he discusses city traffic problems and refers to "cars" in general, he has in mind not one particular car, but several. He is using the word inclusively and employing what Goldstein termed the "abstract attitude." Inability to use a word in a categorical sense (loss of the ability to propositionalize) is a disturbance in or an impairment of "abstract attitude."

Deficiency in abstract attitude does not connote simply an impairment of general mental capacity but has to do with a disintegration of attitudes which Goldstein described as "qualitative." Such loss, which affects all performance fields to a certain degree, occurs particularly in patients with lesions of the frontal lobe. It has also accompanied lesions of other areas of the cortex, especially lesions of the left hemisphere.

A person unable to deal with abstract ideas is handicapped when approaching problems or situations that require understanding. While a participator in his environmental world rather than an outsider looking upon that world, his thoughts and actions are expressed in terms of his restricted personality as it relates to that environment. Since he thinks of concrete objects from an aphasic viewpoint, it is next to impossible for him to use the normal way of planning or making choices, or to think through a problem ideationally to determine cause and effect. To meet emergencies or plan a course of action by relating one aspect of a problem to another, or to explain his own behavior, is extremely difficult.

That is why from the standpoint of abstract behavior some patients seem more disturbed than others. Under careful study, aphasics who appear normal in behavior may reveal much impairment in conceptual thinking. Goldstein[2] stated: "They appeared more stereotyped and reserved—lacked initiative and spontaneity." He further observed that patients disturbed in abstract attitude "fail equally in familiar

[2] Goldstein, Kurt: *Language and Language Disturbances.* Grune & Stratton, Inc., New York, 1948, pp. 5–9.

situations or in new ones which demand the abstract attitude." However, they cope adequately with new tasks when an abstract attitude is not demanded by the situation. When performing concrete tasks, their activities show a more passive compulsive character; they are more stereotyped and rigid. The patient tends to lack drive and spontaneity. His actions appear restrained.

These behavior reactions were observed in patient Dr. S. Impairment of abstract attitude was a major problem of this 68-year-old physician. He could converse happily and easily on golf but became completely lost when the subject was changed to football. Upon beginning therapy he was reluctant to come by himself to the therapist's office but as he became familiar with the surroundings, decided to come alone and traveled by cab from his home to the medical building. Although he appeared oriented in the building (he could go to the second floor alone), it was difficult for him to explain how to get to the therapist's office. If the elevator operator was not aware that he had to get off at the second floor, he had difficulty in requesting "two." Counting from 1 to 100 in series never was difficult for him, providing someone started the series. Embarking on the series of his own volition was impossible. Interrupted in the process of counting, he became blocked and unable to continue with the series. He also had difficulty in starting again. In addition, he was unable to change easily from one type of sequence to another (i.e., from counting numbers to naming months of the year). However, when given the word *January*, he could name the entire monthly series easily.

Under the stress of emotion (i.e., in emotional speech), he often uttered words and sentences which exhibited no speech defect, but when he tried to talk spontaneously in a composed, conversational manner, the naming of concrete objects which required ability in abstract attitude caused him much difficulty in word-finding.

Giving him only the initial sound of a word (not the entire word) was usually of little or no help. He compensated for this impairment by using circumlocutions and paraphrases. Such symptomatology is characteristic of the amnesic aphasic whose primary difficulty is an impaired functioning in higher mental levels—the inability to think symbolically and to assume a conceptual viewpoint or abstract attitude.

We find a patient's abilities in abstract attitude can be effectively evaluated with the Goldstein-Gelb Color Sorting Test, the Goldstein Stick Test, the Goldstein-Sheerer Cube Test, the Weigl Color Form Sorting Test, and the Goldstein-Gelb Object Sorting Tests. These materials may be secured from the Psychological Corporation, 522 Fifth Avenue, New York City. (For their detailed description, see Goldstein's *Language and Language Disturbances*, pages 152–70 [Grune & Stratton, Inc., New York, 1948].) In addition, the Tashkis, Cushman, and Landis printed card test can be used to check sorting ability. We also find that the Bourdon test for measurement of attention, when modified to fit a patient's needs, can be used to test abstract attitudes.

Having determined whether or not the patient has an impairment of abstract attitude, make a careful analysis of the speech and language disturbances and classify as to major type. (See Chapter IV, "Symptomatology.") When deciding upon techniques to be used in resolving the individual's difficulties, try to identify the apraxic areas. Discover in what areas he can or cannot marshal his muscles motorically. (In apraxia, even though paresis is not present, a patient may still be unable to make muscles function as he desires.)

For making a thorough speech and language appraisal, we feel that the Halstead-Wepman test is especially valuable since it permits all required areas to be explored in a single testing session. We also find that the Goldstein Special Examinations for Defects in Language are helpful in testing aphasics. (For details of this testing see Kurt Goldstein's *Language and Language Disturbances*, pages 182–88 inclusive.)

We suggest the Wechsler-Bellevue test not only because it is an excellent performance test, but also because it can give some evidence of pretraumatic as well as posttraumatic intelligence. We feel that no aphasic—or *any* brain-injured individual—should be appraised on the basis of an intelligence test requiring the use of speech and language (e.g., Stanford-Binet). How can he adequately reveal basic abilities on such a test when he has inadequate means with which to express himself?

With some aphasics we also use the Tiegs and Clark Progressive Achievement Tests (E. W. Tiegs and W. W. Clark, Progressive Achievement Tests, California Testing Bureau, Hollywood, California, 1943), because they aid in appraising the reading, writing, spelling, and arithmetical capacities of the patient. From observations made with these tests, one can arrange therapeutic devices on the level of the patient's particular needs.

2. *After Recovery*

We believe that validated psychological tests can and should be used to determine the patient's performance capacity in actual life situations before releasing him from therapy. This data is helpful in aiding a person to select future work or social outlets. The exact time when he is able to follow an old or seek a new pursuit can be determined only by his individual condition. If he has been long under treatment, he may have developed neurotic attitudes.

Most patients eagerly desire to return to their former situations. While we always attempt to help the patient accomplish this, if at all possible, it frequently happens that he would actually be better in some new occupation. Such a conclusion must be presented to the patient most carefully and tactfully. Psychological factors are more important with these recovered aphasics than with most people. Conditions in the home from which he came, personal attitudes toward former work or superiors—all have a bearing on his future success in the economic or social life of his community.

CHAPTER VI

SPEECH AND LANGUAGE PROGNOSIS

"JUST MAKE THE PATIENT AS COMFORTABLE AS POSSIBLE AND try to keep him contented. We may have to institutionalize him but, meanwhile, don't expect him to show much improvement." These well-meaning suggestions have for decades been made by competent medical people. Today such more or less pessimistic recommendations no longer need be made because trained therapists actually are helping a large number of aphasic individuals.

Naturally the premorbid psychological, intellectual, and educational backgrounds, the age and general health of the patient, the site and severity of the cerebral insult are all major factors in determining speech and language prognosis of the aphasic. These may indicate that recovery will be slow and long delayed. Nevertheless, the patient *can* benefit from expert guidance.

Individuals with severe brain injuries (such as gunshot wounds) are usually amenable to therapy. The prognosis for certain cases of apoplexy is also comparatively good. Generally speaking, however, patients with head injuries or brain tumors respond better to retraining than do those with cerebrovascular difficulties. For success in any of these cases, whether arising from trauma or apoplexy, much effort, patience, and skill are required on the part of the therapist if satisfactory recovery is to be achieved.

The authors concur with Goldstein and Wepman in observing that so-called "younger" patients (those under the age of 50) usually have a better chance for recovery than patients in the old-age groups. However, it is not unusual for those in the older brackets to make a fairly good recovery. Patient Jim, 57-year-old tire dealer, was blackjacked by a bandit. The aftermath was a combined disorder of pure motor aphasia with apraxia of the speech muscles. His eight-months-postmorbid vocabulary consisted of the one word, *no*. Today he has a speech vocabulary of over a thousand words. Recently he passed the comprehensive California state examination for renewal of his driver's license.

A patient (whom we call Bob) who was stricken at 58 by a cerebrovascular accident had a problem of amnesic aphasia accompanied by visual agnosia. After a year and a half of concentrated aphasia therapy, Bob resumed his premorbid occupation as a machinist. He carries on limited conversations with fellow workers, answers the telephone as needed, and reads with understanding newspaper headlines or the comic strips.

On the whole, the expressive aphasic has a better chance for recovery than does a receptive aphasic. The probable reason is that an expressive aphasic can more or less appraise what he is attempting to say while the receptive aphasic with a severe auditory and/or visual agnosia is handicapped in determining the merit or quality of his speech and language. Agnosia (particularly auditory agnosia) is usually a difficult problem for the therapist. Auditory agnosia may be resolved in a few weeks with one patient while another may require several months to a year or more of therapy. And in the case of a third patient, recovery may be impossible to achieve.

Improvement in an auditory agnosia patient (or a patient with any type of agnosia) depends greatly upon the functioning capacities retained in his other sensory areas. A loss of recognition in one area (e.g., auditory) necessarily means that other avenues (visual and tactile) must be employed for progress to be made. The individual who suffers from auditory agnosia may also have visual and/or tactile agnosia, and this markedly handicaps recovery of speech and language.

Similarly, the patient with visual agnosia and extensive damage in the auditory area offers a comparatively poor prognosis. Should he also be handicapped in the tactile area, prognosis becomes poorer than if the damage were confined to the visual field.

Prognosis usually is better for visual or tactile agnosia than it is for auditory agnosia. The person who cannot hear nor comprehend what he is saying is markedly handicapped when trying to appraise his speech errors. If all three areas (visual, auditory, and tactile) are damaged, recovery is next to impossible because the therapist has no avenue by which to approach the patient.

Receptive aphasics rarely improve very much, if at all. Progress seems to come nearly always by little stages. If after much perseverance the therapist finds one type of therapy has failed to bring the desired results, other avenues should be explored before giving up. (See Chapter VIII, "Speech and Language Therapy.")

As with all types of aphasia, prognosis for expressive aphasia depends greatly upon the nature and extent of the cerebral lesion sustained and the degree of efficiency with which the corresponding area of the other hemisphere is functioning. The efficiency of speech developed in these patients depends greatly upon the amount of training received by the other hemisphere prior to the insult. The amount of cooperation between the two hemispheres before the occurrence of a lesion must be ascertained, if possible. This is a major factor which must be taken into consideration in determining any prognosis.

Some cases of the apraxic type of expressive aphasia offer an excellent prognosis. After a patient has reacquired some ability to marshal and guide the speech musculature to form monosyllabic words, his ability to hear will aid in speech rehabilitation. Through practice in using the speech muscles, plus observing and feeling and "hearing" what the speech musculature is doing, he begins to discern the difference between correctly and incorrectly formed words. At this point therapy usually advances more rapidly. Of course, successful therapy is always dependent upon the intellectual capacity of the individual. The more damage to the intelligence through injury, the poorer must be the prognosis.

As for transcortical motor aphasia, prognosis is usually good if the cause can be removed. Such patients seldom make marked improvement in uttering voluntary speech. Should the physiological background reveal that his defect is increasing, the patient may later suffer total motor aphasia and become practically mute for emotional utterances. Where psychic trauma has produced only slight dysfunction of the motor area, the prognosis is excellent. Speech will return following recovery from the shock but the patient ought to receive educational therapy to permit an understanding and insight into the emotional blow suffered by his ego.

Prognosis is poor following central motor aphasia. For example, when the cerebral insult is severe and tissue damage great, therapy is of little or no value except as a means of bringing reassurance to the patient whose feelings of insecurity are almost immeasurable.

The pure motor aphasic often has excellent possibilities for recovery but seldom, if ever, makes what might be termed a *complete* recovery. To the average layman such a patient's speech may seem good, but speech will always involve conscious effort on the patient's part although he may appear to be quite normal. The degree of recovery is dependent upon the amount of restitution of previously built motor speech patterns.

In certain cases of initial motor aphasia, the speech and language problems may be eliminated more or less spontaneously through restitution of the damaged substratum following surgical procedures such as draining of abscesses, removal of splinters, tumors, etc.

Similarly, prognosis may be excellent in the case of an amnesic aphasic when restitution of the atomistic processes takes place. There can be marked improvement in ability to employ the abstract concepts but if restitution fails to occur, progress will be slow.

Recent studies indicate that any possible spontaneous improvement made by the aphasic usually comes during the first half year after occurrence of the traumatic incident.[1] Luria[2] found that two periods usually could be looked for in the recovery of an aphasic. During the first six months after cerebral injury, both temporary and permanent language and personality deviations were observed. In the second six-month period following cerebral insult, only persistent language and personality problems were noted. Wepman's study of 71 patients revealed similar findings.[3]

For more than 20 years we have been observing and working from the therapeutic standpoint with speech and language problems in aphasic patients. Experience indicates that it is not at all unusual for an aphasic to make a remarkable recovery within a few months after cerebral injury. Some recover enough to read, write, and speak adequately but most of them tire easily when performing these tasks. They are forced to expend far more than an average amount of effort in doing so. Most patients who become aware of these factors

[1] Butfield, E., and Zangwill, O.: "Re-education in Aphasia," *J. Neurol., Neurosurg. & Psychiat.*, 9:75–79, 1946.

[2] Luria, Alexander: *Topical Syndromes of Traumatic Aphasia* (unpublished manuscript loaned by Helen Black, literary agent of U.S.S.R., New York). Cited by J. M. Wepman in *Recovery from Aphasia*. The Ronald Press Co., New York, 1951, p. 30.

[3] Wepman, J. M.: *Recovery from Aphasia*. The Ronald Press Co., New York, 1951, pp. 68–82.

and who had stamina and fortitude, compensate by throwing themselves wholeheartedly into speech and language attempts. They develop compulsive-obsessive habits while striving for self-improvement. These habits are exceedingly beneficial in aiding ultimate recovery and the wise therapist encourages their formation.

Immediately after the onset of an injury, no therapist can determine with certainty whether or not an aphasic will experience spontaneous recovery. For instance, a patient entirely without speech may seem completely "hopeless" so far as rehabilitation is concerned, yet this same patient frequently makes a real improvement. The amount of spontaneous recovery and the probable length of time required are always unpredictable, varying from patient to patient, so that it is unwise to wait until the end of the initial six-month period following onset to decide whether sufficient recovery permits instituting aphasia therapy. Clinical experience definitely indicates that therapy ought to begin as soon as possible after cerebral injury if maximal benefits are to be derived.

In cases of hemorrhage, therapy ought to be started as soon as bleeding stops. We have started therapy in cases of embolism or thrombosis within 48 hours after the cerebral insult. Sixty-year-old movie producer Harry suffered a cerebrovascular accident on Friday night. His first session of aphasia therapy came on the following Monday morning, an interview devoted to the appraisal of his problem and a *general* discussion of how the speech and language difficulty might be resolved. Early institution of aphasia therapy aids a patient in developing ego strength and frequently serves as a tremendous "boost" to make him realize something is being done immediately to aid his efforts at recovery.

While certain patients may and often do make spontaneous recoveries, every aphasic ought to have the opportunity for speech and language evaluation (as indicated) during the early days of his illness. Therapy initiated immediately following cerebral injury seems to revive a sense of self-importance. The patient feels he is receiving "special attention" and that others are actually concerned about his recovery.

The relationship between patient and therapist is most important. There must be rapport if the individual's feelings of importance and ego strength are to be built up. When rapport is good, the patient is less likely to brood over his plight, to feel sorry for himself, or to develop emotional blocks against recovery. An aphasic's feelings about himself and his problem are vital factors when determining the prognosis of a case.

The family's attitude is equally important when determining the possibility of a patient's recovery. Relatives may exert every effort to aid him. But when the family regards the patient as "hopeless" and openly discusses placing him in a "rest" home, he tends to think of himself as an "outcast" from society. Naturally he displays irritability, anxieties, and frustrations or withdraws within himself and assumes an attitude of "giving up."

Frequently the aphasia therapist is greeted with remarks like: "All this testing and therapy involves so much time and work. Maybe we can't afford it. Is it worth while?" The answer is that when an aphasic has been helped to make himself understood and his wants known; when he has been aided to adapt comfortably to the environment; even enabled to return to his employment or career or profession, such achievements are worth every effort. That is why we insist that speech and language evaluation is indicated in the case of *every* aphasic, no matter how serious or mild the case may appear to be.

Time after time "hopeless" aphasics have made a comparatively good recovery (depending on the nature and extent of cerebral injury). Whatever an aphasic's lack—whether large or small—the deficiency should be explored and all possible help administered as, if, and when needed.

To conclude, based on our combined experiences of a quarter century, prognosis for the aphasic patient depends upon six major factors:

1. The premorbid psychological, intellectual, and educational backgrounds.
2. The age and general health of the patient.
3. The site and severity of the neurological injury.
4. The institution of therapy as soon as possible after the cerebral insult.
5. The aphasic's will to improve.
6. The attitude of the family toward the patient.

CHAPTER VII

INITIAL THERAPEUTIC CONSIDERATIONS

A. DETERMINING GOALS

A TRUE APHASIC RARELY MANIFESTS CLEAR-CUT LOSS IN JUST one narrow language sphere and his problems are never identical with those of any other individual; hence it is impossible to use identical therapeutic procedures for all cases. The individual's particular problems must be studied, his pre- and postmorbid behavior and specific losses determined, after which the therapist must appraise the areas that remain intact because these undamaged portions of the brain play a vital part in the restitution of function, and in the patient's readjustments.

In addition, the patient's own ego image must be carefully studied. In earlier years of aphasia therapy, the therapist's evaluation of the patient's difficulty and self-concept were considered most important. The therapist set the goals and decided upon the order in which a patient's abilities should be stimulated and re-established. Our experience shows it is far more effective to learn the aphasic's concept of himself, since that appraisal is the paramount factor in determining the therapeutic program.

For example, the area selected by the patient for initial therapy frequently is not the one most defective nor even an area in which the therapist believes it best to begin treatment. In fact, a patient's concept of his primary difficulties may be diametrically opposed to those of the therapist, yet we

strongly feel the best treatment usually begins with the problem over which the patient feels his greatest concern and
considers most thwarting.

Examination may reveal the aphasic's true problem is
word-finding, but the patient may feel the writing of his
own name is most important so therapy should begin with
that. Let him practice writing the name until he can sign a
letter or check, thus ending the humiliation incident to making a cross for his signature. The higher the premorbid social
and educational status of the patient, the greater is the embar-
rassment produced by using X for his name. The aphasic
himself must be treated and therapy adapted to his present-
day needs.

Just what are an aphasic's needs? Does he have physical
limitations? (A common result of cerebral injury is hemiplegia of the contralateral side; e.g., injury in the left side of
the brain manifests itself by paralysis of the right side of the
body.) Is the patient ambulatory? Does he have access to a
hospital or clinic where physiotherapy is available? Can he
come to the therapist's office? Will therapy involve house
calls? All these problems must be considered when planning
the therapeutic program to fit the needs of the specific
individual.

It is highly important that an aphasic have physiotherapy
for any physiological needs. In dealing with paralyzed persons at the Orthopaedic Hospital, Los Angeles,[1] physiotherapy
administered just prior to a speech therapy session was particularly beneficial. The change from nonlanguage to language stimulation has usually been welcomed by patients.

In addition to physiological limitations, consideration
should be given to the patient's psychological problems (see
Chapter IX, "Psychological Aspects of Aphasia Therapy")

---

[1] Hansen, Ruth; Longerich, Edward; and Longerich, Mary: "The Physical
Therapy Approach to Spasticity and Athetosis," *Physiotherapy Rev.*, 27:174–81,
1947.

and his re-educational requirements. All these needs must be kept in mind when determining the therapeutic measures involved. Summed up, an aphasic must be regarded as a person functioning in a specific environment and his individual needs considered in the light of what may be necessary to develop him "toute d'une piece."

Since most aphasics fail to recognize all their various inabilities, therapist and patient ought to plan the retraining program together. While discussing proposed therapy with a patient, tactfully explain that although he may fall short of perfection in speech production, the steps you can help him take will make his speech more understandable and acceptable so he can participate effectively in his environment. This explanation requires tact and real ingenuity on the part of the therapist but it can produce amazing results.

Goal recognition is a vital part of aphasia therapy. Both patient and therapist must understand why they are working together and toward what general goals they are striving. If the various aphasia examinations indicate that it is practically impossible for a patient to eliminate certain aphasic symptoms, the therapist must aid that patient to select goals which will permit a comfortable adjustment to his difficulties. These goals must never be so difficult as to doom the patient to utter failure but they should be specific and exact and barely within the reach of the patient. Not only should general goals be set up but there ought to be subgoals which may be achieved within the limits of his frustration tolerance. The attaining of simple goals at frequent intervals boosts the patient's morale and causes him to exert more effort.

At each session (preferably four or five times a week) the therapist should aid the patient to determine his goals. As these are won, both clinician and patient should discuss and recognize the attainments, always with the intention of arousing a sense of pride and victory in the patient. Furthermore, *every* therapeutic session should close on a successful note. Never end a therapy consultation on an unsuccessful note. See that your patient leaves the consultation room aware of his accomplishments during that session. Give him hearty approval as he departs, mentioning with definite assurance the next session "when you'll do even better."

B. Work Habits

Our experience teaches that an aphasic functions most adequately when intent on the task at hand. For this reason, relaxation exercises are not indicated during the therapy session. To keep telling your patient to relax is not only distracting but upsets him. Assume a calm friendly attitude, never showing concern or anxiety if he has difficulty in responding. Constantly but tactfully prod him on to the task at hand.

In severe cases, most patients respond best when trying to perform taxing drills. Confronted with an extremely difficult task, an aphasic exerts real effort and no other approach enables him to do so well. Carefully devised taxing drills develop in the patient a habit of deliberate approach to goals. The development of compulsive-obsessive work habits is strongly recommended in early stages of aphasia therapy. The degree of difficulty of the drill must be planned and adapted to the individual so that even though he concentrates, your patient can barely succeed. He should be kept striving and struggling with the problem while you reassure him that the task is one he can accomplish.

C. Individual Therapy

With aphasics the most rapid progress is made through individual therapy. Formal retraining has to be specifically adapted to a patient's individual needs. The actual retraining takes place in the consultation room where there are no external stimuli to frustrate or distract. As abilities and skills are reacquired, he usually attempts to apply these in everyday situations. Group singing can be of distinct value at this point. Where the majority of the group are normal, i.e., nonaphasic individuals, the singing activity is helpful because it permits an aphasic to feel inconspicuous so that he can try to emulate the normal singers without becoming self-conscious.

In passing, it might be mentioned that we have found it helpful for aphasics to meet in the therapist's reception room. These brief meetings are stimulating and frequently encourage a particular individual to further effort, especially when an extremely crippled aphasic encounters some patient who has made remarkable recovery. Such an experience usually motivates markedly a recently traumatized individual just embarking on his retraining program. Examples are the various meetings of our patients Dr. S. and Eldon, and Mack and Geraldine (see pages 18 and 85).

D. Type of Materials

Where speech is the area receiving primary therapeutic consideration, we begin the treatments with the naming process. The first words taught should aid that patient to adapt to his environment and to maintain biological and psychological equilibrium. Select words which pertain to his tastes, interests, personal biases, hopes, ambitions, sensitivities, and life routine in general.

Suggestions as to therapy procedures recommended here have proved helpful to a great number of patients over the years. Bear in mind, however, that every therapeutic device or scheme used with aphasics must be selected on the basis of an individual patient's intelligence, needs, desires, likes, and interests. The therapist must continually encourage that patient to want help. All materials chosen should elicit and hold his interest. When any procedure fails, other methods should be tried until suitable ones are found. In most cases, many techniques will be used before the desired goals are attained.

Because therapy varies so markedly with each individual patient, specific suggestions as to materials to be used must be limited. Other sections of this book will indicate additional materials for use in therapy.

E. Rapport with Patient

During initial therapeutic sessions the clinician must take every possible step to establish strong rapport with the patient. Without that, little can be accomplished to recover an aphasic's lost abilities. While establishing rapport, point out to your patient that if he seeks help merely because some member of the family desires it, therapy will be more or less futile. He himself must sincerely desire to solve the problem; otherwise your efforts will be of little avail.

This relationship or rapport differs markedly from that which exists between a surgeon and his patient. In the surgeon-patient relationship, the major job is that of the surgeon whose skill is the primary factor in a successful operation. In the aphasia clinician-patient relationship, the clinician also must be highly skilled but this factor is insufficient unless the patient exerts powerful efforts to aid himself. As a therapist, never infer that the patient can solve his problem unaided. Aphasia therapy is definitely a cooperative process where clinician and aphasic work side by side as co-partners in a joint enterprise. Hence the clinician's association with the patient and his family must be friendly. Without cooperation from all concerned, there is little hope of success with the client.

The therapist's attitude toward the patient and his family must always be cordial, but objective. It is futile and time-wasting to sympathize with a patient lest we encourage masochistic enjoyment in his failure. The development of empathy is the real goal.

When handling "stroke" patients, most families deal with the loved one as though he were a child. This attitude only complicates the problem by promoting dependency. When an individual wants help, he should receive it; but when he shows independence and indicates a desire to do for himself, he ought to be permitted so to do. He may lack understandable speech but he is *not* a child and he knows it. Dealing with him as such only creates resentment and hostility. These naturally impede and hinder any drive toward recovery. Patients thus frustrated by some domineering attendant or relative often develop a stubborn attitude and refuse to cooperate, or spend an entire session sulking and pouting. Thereafter, several sessions may be needed to deal with this "resistance" (negative transference) and enable the patient to find some alternative defense against these domestic pressures before we can re-establish rapport and empathy sufficient for therapy.

Our experience teaches that whatever motivates a patient toward recovery is good if it is ethical, honorable, kindly, and decent. Whatever lessens such goal-striving is improper, unwise, and poor therapy, regardless of the thought behind it and regardless of the alleged authority of the person devising the therapy program.

F. Nurse's Attitude toward Patient

The nurse who cares for an aphasic must have some knowledge of the therapeutic goals set up for such patients. In general these are:

1. To develop understandable speech.
2. To develop reading, writing, and spelling skills.
3. To provide opportunities for self-expression.
4. To aid patient to accept himself in the light of his present situation.
5. To aid patient to develop emotional balance.
6. To avoid creating any situation which might cause an anxiety attack.

In striving toward these goals, the following suggestions will be helpful to the nurse who heeds them:

1. Be relaxed and calm around the patient. Try to keep him happy and contented with himself and his surroundings. Avoid forcing him to do things.

2. Avoid making any issue as to his lack of speech. Always phrase your questions so the patient may answer with a "yes," "no," or nod of the head. In some instances a patient indicates "yes" when he actually means "no," and vice versa.

3. Anticipating what the patient is trying to say by voicing it for him markedly impedes progress in speech and language development. Always encourage the patient to speak and do for himself but never make *an issue* over his doing it. If he can read, encourage him to read the newspaper; if he can write his name, encourage him to sign his name rather than make a cross for his signature. Let him take care of his grooming and his physical needs as much as possible. Being allowed to do things for himself aids the patient to build self-respect.

4. Accept an aphasic patient *as he is.* Let him express himself freely on his own speech and language level. Exert every effort to understand what he is trying to tell you—whether it be in words, distorted syllables, or pantomime.

5. If patient swears or voices emotional utterances, *avoid any show of disapproval.* To express annoyance or reprove a patient only inhibits his attempts at communication and may cause withdrawal "into his shell." He will then avoid all efforts to speak.

6. Avoid all discussions pertaining to "before" or "after" his accident, injury, stroke, etc., and never mention his speech inabilities.

7. Avoid putting pressure on a patient to get him to utter

a complete sentence. If he says only the essential words (e.g., nouns, pronouns, and action verbs), show pleasure over such speech efforts. Brief utterances made during early posttraumatic days are most acceptable efforts and they should be praised.

8. When handing patient an object such as a fork, repeat the word *fork* several times. Say it in a confident modulated voice—never with a rising questioning inflection. Similarly, when bathing any part of the patient's body, say the name of that part several times as you wash it. At first, name the parts of the body he can see during the bath (e.g., *arm, hand, leg, foot, toe,* etc.). Later, use such words as *back, ear, head, face, chin,* etc. Use only one-syllable words at first, then two-syllable words such as *shoulder, elbow,* etc.

9. Should patient indicate a desire to be helped with a word, pronounce it slowly and distinctly. Avoid saying, "Watch me as I say it" or "Put your tongue here or there," or the like. Directions regarding correct use of speech musculature are handled by the therapist during the therapy session. Most therapists will discuss and demonstrate to the attendant what can be done to help the patient, especially if he requests such assistance.

10. When the patient seems unable to say a certain word or phrase or cannot perform a given task, *avoid showing concern.* Suggest that he do something else you feel he can do. If he indicates a dislike to try another activity, help him to complete the first task. *Never* reprimand, scold, or tease patient because he is unable to carry out an activity.

11. If a patient tries to tell you something and you can't understand him, suggest by word and pantomime that he draw a picture of what he is trying to say.

12. When patient shows fatigue, suggest a change of activ-

ity or a rest—depending on the degree of fatigue. However, avoid negative suggestions such as, "You're tired now; let's do something else." Avoid all reference to fatigue, anxiety, or tension. Simply intersperse activity with rest periods. Avoid overstimulating the patient. Never suggest too much rest, for that may cause anxiety, withdrawal, and loss of initiative.

13. Avoid discussing with the patient problems pertaining to his family or friends or other patients in the hospital. Those problems are *not* his concern. The aphasic's primary problem is *himself*—his handicaps and his needs.

14. Take advantage of patient's feeling of euphoria (sense of well-being) even though he may have a serious disability. Patient's lack of concern about his condition in the early postmorbid days can be used to motivate constructive habits for speech and language therapy activities and for physical and occupational therapy. Never discuss euphoria as such with the patient, because this is his defense (by denial) against unconscious anxiety.

15. Try to meet all accidents on the part of the patient in a relaxed manner. For instance, make no issue of his spilling food on his robe or tipping over a glass of water. Strive always to establish and *keep* rapport with your patient. Perhaps a comment like "Accidents do happen," accompanied by a real smile will help him to feel less ashamed in the difficult situation.

16. Never make any issue about practicing speech, writing, etc., because suggestions for practice should come from the patient.

17. When helping the patient review material in his speech notebook, make certain that the review session ends on a *successful* note. Closing the practice period with an unsuccessful attempt depresses the patient and impedes progress.

18. Avoid saying "Now relax—and then you say it." (Suggestions for relaxation are often helpful to a spastic, athetoid, or polio patient but not with an aphasic.) To tell the aphasic to relax is distracting and upsetting. You may even precipitate an anxiety attack. Assume a calm friendly attitude and avoid any show of concern or anxiety when he has difficulty in responding.

19. When helping the patient with his speech review, see that *no one* else is in the room. Extraneous stimuli are most distracting to the aphasic.

20. It was explained to the patient during the first therapy session that speech progress will require time and effort. It is necessary for the patient to recognize and accept these factors; otherwise, he tends to become even more discouraged about his aphasia problem. The less said about the time and effort involved, the better. Above all, avoid remarks like "You'll be well in just a short time," etc., because these lead to disillusionment.

21. The patient continually needs help in recognizing his major goals, his subgoals, and his day-to-day goals. These will frequently be discussed with the patient during therapy sessions. As these day-to-day goals are reached, it will aid him if you commend his progress. Such recognition aids him in further goal-setting and attainments.

22. All new words are presented in the therapy sessions. *Never* (especially in early stages of therapy) permit patient to write a word without saying it aloud. The word must be written and spoken as one unified process.

23. Avoid all mention of spelling. That problem is resolved automatically as patient learns to write and say the word. If he attempts to spell aloud, just suggest: "Let's write and say it."

24. Suggest various pastimes for the patient. Do this even

while he is still bedridden. Select activities in which you are confident the patient can be successful and participate *with* him in the activity. For example, if a woman patient starts a knitting project, the nurse should knit, too. By continually motivating a patient to constructive, worth-while activities, you are helping him to avoid self-destructive behavior such as withdrawal and depression.

25. Familiarize yourself with various aspects of the patient's behavior. Study them in the light of his speech and language problems. Keep in mind that the patient is *not* a "different" person because he has aphasia. He is just reacting to his environment in the light of his present difficulties. For suggestions in dealing with various types of personalities, read, study, and use the suggestions found in such books as *Strategy in Handling People* by Webb and Morgan. (See Bibliography, pages 169–74, for similar references.)

26. These suggestions are directed primarily to the nurse, for she is the one who will be spending the most time with the patient. Actually, every member of the hospital staff who has any dealings with the patient— doctor, interne, speech pathologist, psychologist, physiotherapist, occupational therapist—all must cooperate in the speech and language therapy program in order that the patient may derive the maximal benefit. Later, when the family takes over the major responsibility of daily care of the patient, they must unite their efforts in carrying out the therapeutic program.

CHAPTER VIII

SPEECH AND LANGUAGE THERAPY

A. RECEPTIVE APHASIA

I. *Therapy for Visual Agnosia:* As pointed out in the section on Speech and Language Symptomatology, the visual agnosia patient may be disturbed in recognizing physical activities such as running, jumping, laughing, etc. He sees an object or activity but seems unable to name what is seen. When he sees a dog, he is unable to associate the animal with the word *dog* and can't say *dog*. By actual experience we have found single association techniques inadequate in handling the problem of naming objects or "word-naming." We find visual agnosias usually progress more rapidly when the Pavlovian technique (e.g., looking at the object and naming it aloud) is used with combined speaking-writing-reading procedures. In this multiple association technique, the patient must *see* the object, *hear* the spoken name of the object as a unified process, learning to recognize both the written and printed (or typed) word symbol for the object (or action). *Four realms* of learning must be employed: *seeing, hearing, speaking, writing*. (See steps 1–20, pages 110–18.)

The following therapeutic techniques for word-naming have been highly successful with many patients. Through their use the patient not only develops ability in word-naming but is also being trained in reading and writing skills.

A. *Therapeutic Procedures for Word-naming:*

1. Seat the patient in front of a large mirror. Sit beside or slightly behind him. Point to your right or left eye and speak the word *eye*, exaggerating your lip movements. Open your mouth widely as you say *eye*.

   Note that *eye* is said in isolation. Never use it in a sentence during this initial phase of therapy. Later, sentences are excellent devices for therapy. (See steps 27, 30, and 31, pages 121, 122–23.) Utter *eye* with certainty and finality, employing a circumflex or downward inflection. Never use a questioning upward inflection.

   As you speak the word, touch your index finger to the corner of your left eye. Repeat this activity several times before suggesting that the patient imitate this movement. If necessary, take his index finger and place it at the corner of his left eye. As the finger touches the skin, patient and therapist say *eye*.

   If he has difficulty with this procedure, avoid any show of concern. Instead, smile and encourage him to continued attempts, accepting every effort he makes. Avoid all mention of inaccuracies in articulation or grammar. Patient Joe, long before his cerebral insult, had customarily said *morneg* for *morning* and *he don't* for *he doesn't*. No attempt was made to correct these errors. The important concern was to aid him in re-establishing communication and to help him make known his wants so he could adapt to his social world.

   Avoid working too long during one session on word-naming exercises. When the patient shows fatigue or diminishing interest, shift your therapeutic activities. Be sure to end each therapy session on a successful note. Deliberately go over again some test which he can successfully handle—then stop the session.

2. Prepare for the patient a "picture-object notebook." Use white, unlined, 8½ × 11 in. loose-leaf paper. Apply alphabetical stickers so pages may be indexed. Paste or draw a picture of a human eye at the top of a page; then with a colored pencil or crayon write or print the word *eye* in large cursive letters on the lower half of the page. (With aphasics who know only how to print, the word should be printed.)

3. Next say *eye* as you simultaneously trace the word with the index finger of your hand. Utter the word as you write the downstroke of the first *e*. Extend the utterance of the word until it is completely traced.[1]

4. Hold the patient's writing hand, assisting him to trace, and say the word *eye* over and over until he seems capable of emulating step 3.

5. After he has traced the word several times as in step 4, suggest that he tell you (by nod, for example) if he will try to write and say the word without looking at the book. If he agrees, close the picture-object notebook so he cannot see the picture-object or word. Have him start at the upper left-hand corner of a separate sheet of paper, writing and saying *eye* as outlined in steps 3 and 4. Should he err in writing or printing, do *not* let him cross out or erase the mistakes, for this is only confusing to the patient. Let him have another sheet—"hide" sheet—to place over the incorrect attempt. Now have him open the picture-object notebook to trace and say the word *eye*. Continue this tracing activity until he indicates

---

[1] Quintilian advocated that learning the sound and *form* of the letter should be one unified process. Seneca recommended that the teacher place his hand on the pupil's hand to guide his fingers in writing.

readiness to write and say the word. Then let him write and say the word accurately without looking in the notebook.

If the patient's problem involves mirror writing or mirror printing, direct him to start at the extreme upper left-hand side of the page and move from left to right.

An aphasic who prints his letters may have difficulty making downward strokes in letters like *l* in *log*, *t* in *top*, *k* in *rock*, *r* in *rat*, *h* in *hand*. He may initiate individual letters from right to left rather than from left to right. For example, in the case of patient John, age nine,[2] he printed ʃʃʅ in *man*, rather than Ꮽ ; instead of starting *m* with the initial downstroke, he began at the right with an upward stroke. He made a similar mistake in printing *n* and crossed his *t*'s from right to left.

When demonstrating to such a patient, always use whole words (not individual or printed letters) and show him how to print on the downward stroke moving from left to right. For example:

boy	hand	mamma	bun
car	pig	man	van
dog	jar	queen	water
ear	rock	sack	box
fan	ball	rat	zoo

6. A second picture notebook similar to the picture-object notebook should be prepared. (See step 2.) Paint or draw on the first page a human eye identical

[2] Aphasia may occur in children as well as adults. However, it is much more difficult to detect aphasic problems in children.

to that in the picture-object notebook. Leave the remainder of the page blank. Have patient look at the picture; then follow suggestions in steps 4 and 5; write and say the word *eye*.

7. Proceed with the word *ear* just as you did with the word *eye* in steps 1–6.

8. Rule an unlined, 8½ × 11 in. sheet of paper into approximately 16 to 20 squares. Scatter the written or printed words *eye* and *ear* over the page, then ask the patient to read them aloud. If there are any difficulties, return to steps 3 and 4.

9. Proceed as in step 8. But instead of using the written or printed words *eye* and *ear*, type these in the squares.

10. Let patient file the object sheets *eye* and *ear* under the "E" section of his notebook. (See step 2.) This is the only suggestion we ever make regarding letters.

11. Proceed with the words *nose* and *mouth* as outlined in steps 1–9.

12. Prepare a reading (longhand or printed) sheet for the four words *eye*, *ear*, *nose*, and *mouth*. (See step 8.)

13. Prepare a typed reading sheet for the four words *eye*, *ear*, *nose* and *mouth* and proceed as in step 9.

14. Using the picture-object notebook, let the patient see a picture and then name it. If difficulty is encountered, return to steps 1–5. Then have him repetitiously point to specific parts of his own body and name each organ at the moment his finger touches the object:

   a. eye   c. nose
   b. ear   d. mouth

Should he falter in naming body parts, return to steps 1–5. Note that words in the above series are related to each other as components of the lost "body image." When learning a word series, it helps the patient when he says the words in a sort of rhythmic fashion. The series should be practiced several times daily so it will not be forgotten. (See steps 1–9.)

15. Following steps 1–14, present additional word series to the patient; i.e.:

a. arms	c. legs
b. hands	d. feet

16. Proceeding as in steps 1–14, present the following words:

a. head	a. chin
b. hair	b. cheek

Some patients tend to confuse words like *head* and *hair*. In such cases, practice persistently on the word *head* until patient can easily write and say it in unison with you. Do likewise with the word *hair*. Next, have him alternate writing and saying the two words *head* and *hair* until he executes each word accurately. Proceed similarly with the series *chin*, *cheek*.

17. Note that up to this point only monosyllabic object words have been used. We find it best that 10 or 15 monosyllabic words should be thoroughly learned before trying two-syllable words. This enables the patient to develop the concept while uttering the word simultaneously with his tracing. Next, proceed with a two-syllable word such as *mother*. If he has always addressed his mother as "mama," use that word.

18. In uttering the word *mother*, use procedures outlined in steps 1–15. Speak the first syllable, *mo*, just

as the downstroke of *m* is made. Extend the utterance of the *o* until patient is ready to trace the second syllable, *ther*. *Ther* is uttered just as the downstroke of *t* is made. Draw out the syllable *ther* in utterance until *r* is completely traced.

19. Use the procedures described in steps 10–17 to develop additional word series as shown below:

a. mother	a. shirt	a. ham
b. baby	b. trousers	b. eggs
c. milk	c. socks	c. toast
d. bottle	d. shoes	d. coffee
	e. tie	
	f. hat	
	g. coat	

Continue with this activity until patient has at least 50 to 75 words in his concrete object vocabulary. Further suggestions for words to be learned are:

CONCRETE NOUNS——ONE SYLLABLE

ax	bird	cane	cuff
back	boat	cap	cup
bag	bow	car	dart
ball	bowl	cart	deer
bat	boy	chair	desk
bead	bread	clock	dime
bean	broom	cloud	dish
bear	brush	comb	dog
bed	bug	corn	dome
bee	bull	cot	door
beef	cab	cow	dove
beet	calf	crab	drape
bell	cake	cream	dress
belt	can	crow	drum

CONCRETE NOUNS—ONE SYLLABLE (*Continued*)

duck	key	pants	sea
face	king	paw	seed
fire	kit	pea	shelf
fish	kite	peach	shell
fist	knee	pear	ship
foot	knife	pen	sink
fork	knit	pie	sky
frog	lamp	pig	snow
girl	lark	pill	soap
glass	leaf	pin	soup
goat	light	plane	spade
golf	lip	plow	spoon
goose	log	plum	star
grape	lunch	pole	stool
grass	lungs	prune	stove
gum	man	puff	suit
gun	mat	pump	sun
heart	match	queen	tack
heel	meat	rag	tea
hen	mill	rain	tent
hill	mit	rat	throat
hip	moon	rice	thumb
hoe	moth	ring	tire
hog	mud	road	toad
horse	mule	robe	toe
hose	nail	rock	tongue
house	neck	roof	tooth
hut	nest	room	tree
ice	net	rope	truck
ink	nut	rose	tub
jam	oar	rug	vase
jar	pail	salt	vest
jaw	pan	sauce	wall

CONCRETE NOUNS—ONE SYLLABLE (*Continued*)

watch	wheat	wife	wood
weed	wheel	wing	wrist

CONCRETE NOUNS—TWO SYLLABLES

ankle	dinner	jelly	pony
apple	doctor	lemon	rabbit
apron	donkey	lettuce	razor
arrow	engine	lily	sugar
bowling	eyebrow	lion	supper
breakfast	eyelid	mamma	table
brother	father	ocean	tiger
butter	feather	olive	turkey
candle	finger	orange	walnut
cigar	gravy	pencil	water
circus	hammer	pepper	window
daddy	honey		

Never use nonsense words. Our clinical experience indicates they are utterly useless to the patient. The more sincere his desire for rehabilitation, the more annoyed he becomes when drilled with nonsense syllables.

We like to supply the patient with concrete words from his current environment. Explore all major pretraumatic interests and select from those areas concrete nouns to aid in developing his naming vocabulary. Ask the family and associates as to life areas about which he was most enthusiastic prior to trauma. As progress comes, use words in the everyday experience of the patient. Proceed with these series as per steps 1–17. With 30 to 40 words in his object-naming vocabulary, the patient may tend to change his procedure in correcting errors. Instead

of returning to the picture-object notebook and re-
tracing the word, he may want to look at his model
(written in colored pencil or crayon). Should this
method bring good results, omit the tracing step in
the correcting phase of learning words. Always let
your patient make this decision, however.

20. Practice each word series until it becomes an automatic procedure for the patient. Later, when he
wishes to produce the name of an object, direct him
to say aloud the appropriate series and stop when the
needed word is recognized.

Only really serious cases adhere long to this
method of word-naming concrete nouns. Most patients will produce audible symbols for objects without using a word series as soon as they can. Each is
eager to throw away "crutches" and the more you
encourage this desire, the faster recovery is accomplished.

21. Always let the patient work out his own mnemonic
devices. He may discover that words difficult for him
to produce alone are easier to say in certain phrases,
and this discovery gives the needed stimulus. One
physician-patient and a certain surgeon-patient
could easily say *throat* when they preceded it with
the previously learned words *eye*, *ear*, *nose*, and
————. Single words become stimuli for other
words. For instance, after patient Catherine learned
hair, she found that prolonging the *r* sound helped
her start the word *ribbon*. Following acquisition of
the word *eye*, it became easier to say *eyebrow* and
eyelash.

22. Songs are excellent vehicles to bring forth needed
responses. While learning the word *rowboat*, patient
Catherine discovered by singing the song, "Row,
Row, Row Your Boat" in unison with the therapist

she could get the word *row* started. When she began therapy, her spontaneous speech vocabulary consisted of *Hi*, used to address anyone. Sometimes she uttered the word *no*.

Some patients after repeating a verse or song can produce an entire phrase or sentence that was previously impossible. Major-league pitcher John could say *ball game* after singing "Take me out to the ball game." Later, *peanuts* and *crackerjack* were recovered by singing "Buy me some peanuts and crackerjack." The first counting attempts came spontaneously as he continued the song: "It's one, two, three strikes; you're out." John was exceedingly proud of this achievement.

23. Frequently words become easier to understand and remember when given in an appropriate context. For example, before patient Catherine could say *beau*, a mnemonic tie-in was made with the phrase "My husband is my ———." After a few trials, she was able to say *beau*. Mnemonic associations given to a physician-patient were:
   a. Michigan is on the 50-yard *line*.
   b. The baby should drink homogenized *milk*.
   c. He sprained his *ankle*.
   d. We go swimming at the *seashore*.
   e. Hiawatha has a bow and *arrow*.
   f. You have met the king and *queen*.
   g. I like lemon *pie*.
   h. I like to eat bread and *butter*.
   i. Jane is my *wife*.
   j. The directions are north, south, east, and *west*.
   Each mnemonic association above brought forth the desired response.

24. Frequently the Pavlovian approach proves effective in word-finding of concrete nouns, i.e., *nominal*

aphasia. For example, when teaching patient Helen the word *water* it was presented on a particularly warm day. As she entered the consulting room, the therapist remarked, "It's so warm. Wouldn't you like a glass of cold water?" Helen nodded because she had not yet learned to say *yes.* As the glass was handed to her, the therapist said *water.* Each time Helen raised the glass to her lips, the therapist repeated *water.* After seven repetitions of this activity, the patient voluntarily said *water.* This procedure was repeated three times during the therapy session. By the end of the hour Helen had made several excellent utterances of the word.

Similarly, a cup of coffee was used to help another physician-patient reacquire the word *coffee.* Other Pavlovian techniques used were as follows:

a. Have patient match picture and word cutouts. (Picture-and-word-matching cards may be secured from Milton Bradley Company, Springfield, Massachusetts.) Teach the patient to say the name of the picture-object as he matches the cutouts.

b. Suggest lotto word games, requiring matching of pictures. As the patient "plays" his picture block on the lotto card, he names the picture-object. Be very careful to select lotto games that are not childish! The authors have found the following types of lotto picture games helpful: Good Things to Eat; Wearing Apparel; Articles of Furniture in the Home; etc.

Of course, it is understood that it is necessary to combine such activities with the procedures described in steps 1–5.

25. When the patient has at least 50 to 75 words in his vocabulary, begin with simple action words such as

run, eat, go, and employ speech-writing combinations as outlined in steps 1–21. Proceed with these verbs until patient has at least 30 to 40 of them in his vocabulary. The following verbs are suggested:

ACTION WORDS

bark	go	row
bite	hide	rub
break	hit	run
climb	hop	shave
close	hug	sing
cry	hunt	ski
cut	jump	slide
dig	kick	smile
dive	lick	stretch
drink	mow	swim
fight	open	swing
fly	ride	throw
fry	rock	walk
give		wash

These may be followed by sensory verbs such as *see, hear, smell, feel, touch,* etc.

26. Proceed similarly as in steps 1–21 with pronoun *I.* This pronoun was taught to patient Ruth by having her point to herself with her index finger. Patient Bill learned *I* when the therapist told him to open his mouth and assume a "Joe E. Brown" smile.

27. Dictate short sentences to patient, using the suggestions in steps 1–26. The following are actual sentences used with a professional man:

I smell.	I enjoy bowling.
I eat toast.	I enjoy golf.
I eat cereal.	

28. Utilizing procedures in steps 1–27, teach the patient short phrases for use in conversation. Patient Barbara's first learned phrase was "Thank you." She immediately employed it in the reception room by saying "Thank you" to the secretary as she handed Barbara her next appointment card. Other suggestions for short conversational phrases are:

Hello.	Good morning.	Yes.
How are you?	Pardon me.	Please.

29. Proceed as in steps 1–19 with the words *open-close*. A book or door can be used for the action of opening and closing.

30. Sometimes it is easier for the patient to learn an action word such as *wash* by using an action sentence like "I wash my hands with soap." In learning this sentence, the physician-patient first unwrapped a bar of soap. Then at the washbowl in the consulting room, he washed his hands. As he rubbed his hands with soap in the water, the therapist and he repeated together, "I wash my hands with soap." When he saw the picture of a person washing his hands, he started his own pantomime of hand-washing which served as the trigger for starting the words *I wash*. Next, the words *wash, hands* (review for him), and *soap* were worked out with speech-reading-writing, as outlined.

    Patient Rita (a young mother) learned the words *rock, baby*, and *arms* by working on the action sentence, "I rock my baby in my arms." Procedure was similar to those described above.

31. Pantomimic actions frequently serve as stimuli for sentences in series. Patient and therapist stand before a mirror. Show him how to shape his hands like field glasses and look through the improvised holes.

Say in unison with therapist "I see with my *eyes*."
As he says the word *eyes*, have him point to eyes as
in step 1. Proceed similarly with ears. Cup hands
over ears and say "I hear with my *ears*." Point to ear
at moment *ear* is spoken. Then continue:

I smell with my nose.	I walk with my legs.
I eat with my mouth.	I kick with my feet.
I stretch with my arms.	

Practice each action series until patient can do it
with ease.

32. Proceed as in steps 1–19 with monosyllabic, then
    bisyllabic adjectives and adverbs. Colors may be
    taught by using mnemonic associations such as
    "Three cheers for the *red*, *white*, and *blue*." "Grass
    is *green*." "Sunkist *oranges*." Granich[3] cites the in-
    cident of the patient who had difficulty in saying
    yellow. After a few repetitions by the therapist of
    " 'Why, you dirty coward,' said Wild Bill, 'you're
    just plain ————,' " the word could be said.

33. Following procedures in steps 1–19, take preposi-
    tions such as *up* and *down*. Point upward as the
    word *up* is said. Point downward as the word *down*
    is said. Take patient's hand and make a definite
    movement up while saying *up* emphatically. Then
    move arm downward with a definite movement and
    say *down*. Patient repeats with therapist until he can
    do it alone. These actual spatial-motor associations
    help him to initiate the utterance of the word.

34. Proceed as in steps 10–18 with additional pronouns,
    interjections, and conjunctions and the "written
    word" numbers *one* to *twenty-five*. In more difficult
    cases, it helps to use bodily actions with such words

[3] Granich, L.: *Aphasia: A Guide to Retraining*. Grune & Stratton, Inc., New
York, 1947, pp. 55–56.

as *oh!* and *ow!* Patient Margaret, by placing her arms in the shape of an *O* as the therapist aided her to round her lips, was taught to say *oh!* As the tips of the fingers came together, the word *oh!* was uttered in a tone of surprise. In teaching patient Harvey to say *ow!*, he was instructed to shrug his shoulders as if a pin had stuck him. This bodily action was the only stimulus needed for the production of the word.

35. Always try to employ words and sentences which may be used as stimuli for other words. The physician-patient found that by attempting to "find" the word *is*, he could start with his name, e.g., Bill, and then come forth with "Jane is my wife." After repeating this sentence, he would stop after saying *is* for he realized it was the word he wanted.

36. Using words in patient's "word-naming–writing–dictation" vocabulary, prepare five- and six-word sentences for him to read. At the next session, present the same sentences typewritten and have him read this material.

37. Using patient's vocabulary, write in longhand incidents or stories for him to read. Present this same material typewritten. For additional helpful material we suggest the following books:

   a. Fernald, Grace M.: *Remedial Techniques in Basic School Subjects* (McGraw-Hill Book Co., New York, 1943).

   b. Lewis, Norman: *How to Read Better and Faster* (Thomas Y. Crowell Co., New York, 1944).

B. *Therapeutic Procedures for Alexia:*

   1. *Therapy for recognition of written or printed words:* Visual agnosics may be disturbed only in recognizing written or printed words. For these patients use therapeutic techniques outlined in steps 1–37 above.

If patient recognizes objects or activities, omit the picture-object notebook (step 6 of Therapeutic Procedures for Word-naming, pages 112–13). Therapies would involve naming, writing, and dictation activities: steps 1–5; 7–37.

2. *Therapy for defect in geometric-optic concept:* When the geometric-optic concept of objects or written and printed words is disturbed, patient may resort to head and eye movements for tracing. Always use the method which proves easiest for him.

   In cases of homonymous hemianopia, Pangle[4] had patient turn the book sideways and read from top to bottom of the pages. He found this method particularly helpful for some of the more difficult cases. We have not made similar observations but believe that the procedure has merit.

3. *Therapy for recognition of numbers:*
   a. Follow procedures as in Therapeutic Procedures for Word-naming, steps 1–37, pages 110–24. Picture-objects used for numbers may be beans, sticks, blocks, or the like. At the top of the first page draw or paste a picture of one block (or bean or stick), then with a crayon or colored pencil write the number *1*. Proceed similarly for all numbers up to 25.
   b. Using these word-naming procedures, steps 1–37, continue with numbers to 100. Most patients need to trace only the first few numbers. The average patient proceeds with number training much more rapidly than when starting training in word-naming. Our experience demonstrates that training in word-naming distinctly helps training in numbers. Since the ability to work out arithmetical problems mentally is greatly

[4] *Ibid.*, p. 59.

dependent on the ability to understand words, training in the reading of words logically comes first.

c. When beginning therapeutic work on the simplest combinations of addition, subtraction, multiplication, division, base procedures entirely on concrete situations applicable to patient's background. Use beans, blocks, sticks, or the like to add, subtract, multiply, and divide. Additional suggestions may be found in Fernald's *Remedial Techniques in Basic School Subjects*, Chapter XIV, pages 213–55 (McGraw-Hill Book Co., New York, 1943).

4. *Therapy for paraphasia:*

a. *Procedures for paragrammatism:*

1[a]. Follow suggestions in Therapeutic Procedures for Word-naming, steps 1–37. Instead of using the picture-object notebook, prepare a word notebook using colored crayons or pencils. This may be called the patient's *speech dictionary*. After one-syllable words are mastered, use two-syllable words such as those listed on page 117. Later three- and four-syllable words may be used, e.g., *elephant, alfalfa, alligator, grandfather, grandmother*, etc.

2[a]. With certain patients it is helpful to make a tape recording of his reading-speaking-writing words, then play this back for his observations and corrections.

3[a]. Frequently we have written a word incorrectly uttered by patient to show the error, but this must be tactfully done to avoid causing frustrations. For some odd reason, patients feel and sense a correct utterance and invariably fail or refuse to notice an error which occurred a few seconds before or after the correctly uttered word.

4ª. Singing helps many patients. An individual often marshals the sounds of a word in correct sequence when he sings or says it in rhythm, whereas he has difficulty in just attempting to say it. In learning the word *baby*, patient Sue was helped when she sang, "Rock-a-bye *baby*."

5ª. Nonsense syllables are valuable only as time-consumers but tongue twisters occasionally help, as shown in the following sentences:

a¹. Polly pruned pears and put them on platters.

b¹. Bobbing bumble bees buzzed—*hummmm hummmm hummmm.*

c¹. Kay kicked catty Katey.

6ª. Counting from 1 to 100 is helpful. Patients frequently can say in series numbers that they cannot marshal correctly in isolation. Patient Gerry said *seben* for *seven* when saying the word in isolation but spoke it correctly when uttering the number as one of a series.

7ª. It has proved of value for patients to "find" small words in long words such as:

ha<u>mm</u>er	under<u>shirt</u>
eye<u>brow</u>	<u>eye</u>lash
wal<u>nut</u>	<u>eye</u>l<u>id</u>
<u>can</u>dle	

b. *Procedures for agrammatism:*

1ª. Follow suggested steps 11–23, 31 for sentences in series. Have patient memorize various groups of sentences so he may become aware of word order:

I see with my eyes.   I stretch with my arms.
I hear with my ears.   I walk with my legs.
I smell with my nose.   I kick with my feet.

I have two eyes.   I have two arms.
I have two ears.   I have two hands.
I have one nose.   I have one mouth.
I have two legs.   I have two feet.

2[a]. Memorize by rote 20 to 25 stock phrases used in conversation; e.g.:

     a[1]. Good morning.
     b[1]. Good evening.
     c[1]. Thank you.
     d[1]. Pardon me.
     e[1]. Goodbye.
     f[1]. How are you?

3[a]. Give patient sentences to complete such as:

     a[1]. I drink (*coffee*, *tea*, or *milk*).
     b[1]. I wash my hands with soap and (*water*).
     c[1]. I sweep with a (*broom*).

4[a]. Ask patient to compose two-word sentences; e.g.:

     write-letter   wash-face
     eat-steak   jump-rope

5[a]. Have patient look at sentences written in mixed word order, then ask him to put words in correct order; e.g.:

"Morning eat I breakfast the in." (I eat breakfast in the morning.)

Then have him write and say the sentence (as described on pages 110–18).

6[a]. Give patient a set of five or six cards. Each card should display one word of a meaningful sentence. Let him place cards in order. This is excellent training in "word order." Follow this activity by having patient write and say the sentence. (See pages 110–18.)

7ᵃ. Perform a particular activity and name the word simultaneously with the movement (e.g., walking, kicking, smiling, etc.). Next, have patient perform the movement as he says the word. Then have him name the action as you execute the movement. Next, point to the patient and say, "You are smiling." Have patient do the same for you. Follow this by the repeating of the sentence, "The boy beat the drum." As each word is said, point to a finger. Let each finger represent one word.

Repeat the sentence three or four times, then suggest that patient point to the fingers on his hand as he says the sentence.

5. *Therapeutic procedures for paragraphia:* When paragraphia occurs in conjunction with agnosia, it is wise to combine therapy with word-naming–dictation activities. To alleviate writing difficulties, follow reading-writing-dictation activities as described in Therapeutic Procedures for Word-naming, steps 1–37, pages 110–24. Again, may we emphasize that learning to copy or write the alphabet is of little or no value to an aphasic, unless association pathways are simultaneously reinforced.

II. *Therapy for Auditory Agnosia:*

A. As in other types of aphasia, always select the subjects most appealing to the patient and explore each to aid him in developing an inner awareness of what is being recorded in his ear. When an avenue of interest does not seem to produce the desired results immediately, do not discontinue it. If patient appears to have been interested in this subject before, then therapy should be more effective here.

Should a specific approach bring good results, the method should be thoroughly exploited. Continue working in this interest area so long as patient's attention can be sustained.

B. After becoming familiar with the interests of a particular patient, plan therapy accordingly. Methodologies will include particularly the employment of visual, tactile, and kinesthetic stimuli—what the patient can see, feel, or taste.

C. Follow suggestions for word-naming in the section on Therapy for Visual Agnosia, steps 1–37, pages 110–24. The making of a picture-object notebook in line with their own interests is particularly interesting and helpful with some patients.

D. The methods described under Therapeutic Suggestions for Apraxia, Therapeutic Procedures for Word-naming, steps 1–57, pages 136–49, prove advantageous with some patients.

E. Patients may be helped by aiding them in the formation of various words. By learning the "feel" of how a sound is made as it is uttered, patient is frequently helped to develop ability in recognizing a spoken word. For this methodology, follow suggestions under Therapeutic Procedures for Word-naming, pages 110–24.

F. Techniques under Therapy for Visual Agnosia, Therapeutic Procedures for Word-naming, may be used in connection with objects producing sound. For example, a *watch* can be presented to a patient who is allowed to see, feel, and hear it tick. Then ask him to write and say aloud *watch*. Repeat this procedure over and over as patient gains ability to use these combined stimuli. Ask him just to feel (not see or hear it), then write and say the word *watch*. Similarly, drill him in hearing the tick of the watch, then writing and saying the word aloud. Other materials for presentation in this way are:

1. whistle
2. horn
3. drum

G. Adapt all these methods to the needs and interests of the individual patient. As outlined for handling amnesic aphasias, pages 155–56, begin auditory agnosia therapy by using concrete objects, then verbs, adjectives, adverbs, etc. See suggestions under steps 1–37, pages 110–24. Individual words should be followed by two-word phrases, three-word phrases, short sentences, etc.

III. *Therapy for Auditory Music Agnosia:* The aphasia therapist must have extensive musical training to be properly qualified to handle these problems. Only by understanding the real needs of such patients can they be approached therapeutically and aided in the rehabilitation of basic musical capacities. Avoid discussing patient's marked losses because these are most frustrating to an aphasic. Therapeutic devices will be similar to those for auditory agnosia. See steps 1–7, pages 110–13, and Chapter VII, "Initial Therapeutic Considerations."

IV. *Therapy for Tactile Agnosia:* Direct therapy for tactile agnosia usually is not indicated in speech and language recovery. If patient can be approached therapeutically through visual and/or auditory realms, it is much easier to employ those avenues in relearning speech and language rather than to attempt to delve into the tactile problem for rehabilitation. See therapeutic suggestions for visual agnosia and auditory agnosia, pages 109–31.

When visual or auditory areas are seriously affected, the tactile functions must be employed to furnish instructional stimuli. For instance, with a visual agnosic, ask him to feel an object, e.g., watch; listen to it tick; listen to the word *watch* as it is uttered; trace around the watch with a pencil to sense its form. Then write and say the word *watch*. Follow suggestions for word-naming under Therapy for Visual Agnosia, pages 110–24. Precede the presentation of each new object word with feeling-tracing activities as described above for the word *watch*. Here tactile stimuli are used as instructional cues for speech and language therapy.

If all three areas—visual, auditory, and tactile—are affected, then tactile agnosia becomes a more serious handicap.

V. *Therapy for Body Agnosia (Autotopnosia, Autotopagnosia, Topagnosia) and Agnosia of Time and Space:*

A. Drilling patient to select his right or left hand, right or left eye, etc., is time-consuming and usually brings little results. It is far better to plan definite activities for a patient. For example, it was suggested to the physician-patient that he go to the roof garden of the hospital for refreshments. Specific directions were given as to left and right turns. He quickly learned to repeat and follow them.

B. We have found it advantageous in handling topagnostic patients to set up actual life situations as exercises. In this way a direct emotional feeling tone and response builds up within the patient. For example, by actually walking about the home or in a hospital ward or corridor on crutches, or with a cane, the patient finds out his relative distance from other patients or from any object in his surroundings. The use of occupational therapy, especially where there are workshops and tools available to the patient, is most beneficial. His own experimenting with tools aids him in the adaptation of his hands to the instrument in the performing of a task. Materials whose surface is rough and thus readily noticed through digital and tactile manipulations augment the recovery of recognition. Wepman,[5] mentions success along the above lines. The point is —we always endeavor to create tasks whose accomplishment tends to reorient the patient with the life he will encounter every day.

C. Drill patient on setting the hands of a clock to aid his relearning how to tell time. To aid patient Betty in judging time, the office secretary wrote on the back of the card the hour Betty was to leave home for the therapist's office. Slowly Betty gained comprehension of the duration and passage of time.

VI. *Therapy for Transcortical Sensory Aphasia:*

A. Follow suggestions for speaking-writing-dictation activities under Therapy for Visual Agnosia, Therapeutic Procedures for Word-naming, pages 110–24.

B. In case of paraphasia, follow suggestions given on pages 126–29.

VII. *Therapy for Abstract Attitude Paraphasia:* Follow procedures outlined for paragrammatism and agrammatism, pages 126–29. Cases of abstract attitude paraphasia are exceedingly difficult from the standpoint of training, and progress is usually slow. Real effort has to be exerted to make any headway. The ability to handle abstract ideas is one of the most complex mental functions and is therefore one of the first to be lost in brain disorders.

[5] Wepman, J. M.: *Recovery from Aphasia.* The Ronald Press Co., New York, 1951, p. 209.

VIII. *Therapy for Hysterical Amblyopia:* In cases of hysterical amblyopia, the outlined procedures for word-finding are practically useless. That problem should be attacked with hypnotherapy, hypnoanalysis, and psychological counseling based on emotional material elicited from the patient.

A. The initial step is to have a thorough examination made by a competent neurologist. The case may involve trauma, narcotics, or true hysteria. It may involve color blindness or narrowed fields of vision. There may be a hitherto unrecognized brain lesion. If diagnosis is definite that the condition is hysteria, hypnotherapy can be most helpful.

B. *Procedures for Hypnotherapy:*

    1. At initial interview, draw out patient tactfully to get his explanation as to when, where, and how he thinks the dimness of vision began. See what *he* believes caused it. Look for strong feelings about or toward some member of his family or someone with whom he works or is associated in daily life. Is he repressing deep feelings of annoyance, anger, shyness, anxiety, boredom, confusion, disappointment, dislike, rivalry, envy, guilt, or fear?

       Is he concealing the still stronger feelings of remorse, rage, disgust, loathing, hate, jealousy, despair, aftereffects of shock, or desires for revenge? Is he filled with sadness, grief, hostility, resentment, shame, surprise about some event, wonder, worry, or does he feel rejected and unwanted? Has he had recurrent dreams or nightmares? Are there any indications that he is a voyeur or has been? Does he think he saw something terrible occur? Has he read any book or seen any movie or show recently which strongly disturbed him? The point is—what is he trying to avoid seeing?

2. Have him lie down but avoid all mention of hypnosis. Stress your desire to help him get relaxed. Most hysterics are excellent subjects and quickly go into fairly deep trance. For induction techniques see the third edition of *Hypnotism Today*, by LeCron and Bordeaux (Grune & Stratton, Inc., New York, 1952). At this session, use only direct suggestive therapy. Spend 30 minutes to an hour on these and be sure to drive home plenty of strong suggestions that he is comfortable, enjoys being relaxed, and is looking forward to seeing you again. Stress strongly that he will now be able to see much more clearly and that his eyes will be in perfect condition hereafter. Before rousing him, suggest that he will relax far more at the next visit, which should be within seven days.

3. At the next session, take 15 to 20 minutes again to draw him out and learn how he feels. See if he thinks his vision has improved. If so, completely repeat step 2 and instruct him to return for a third session.

   If vision hasn't improved, begin hypnoanalysis. For help in this, see: the third edition of *Hypnotism Today*, by LeCron and Bordeaux (Grune & Stratton, Inc., New York, 1952); *Hypnotherapy of War Neuroses*, by Watkins (The Ronald Press Co., New York, 1949).

B. EXPRESSIVE APHASIA

I. *Therapeutic Suggestions for Apraxia:*

A. *Therapeutic Procedures for Word-naming:* The apraxic patient who not only lacks ability to use the speech muscles for speech but cannot use them for *all* purposes must first be taught how these muscles function. For such training any or all of the following activities may be used:

1. Teach him to blow out a candle or a match. You may need to suggest that he heave a big sigh. Always demonstrate exactly what you mean. Often the sigh alone will cause enough exhalation of air to make the flame flicker.

2. Have him blow a feather or a light piece of paper across a smooth surface. Let him see in a mirror how his lips purse when he blows.

3. Place his hand on your larynx. As you pronounce the *a* in *above*, he feels the vibration of the vocal cords. Demonstrate several times and then suggest that he try to do it. Have him feel his own larynx while uttering this sound.

4. Let him listen through a stethoscope to the vibration of your vocal cords when you say *a*. Give several demonstrations and then place the stethoscope button on his larynx while he imitates the procedure.

5. Purse your lips and whistle. This may be difficult for him in early therapy but it is wise to try it at each session. Sometimes the response is amazingly quick and good. Each slightest success in beginning therapy means much to the apraxic.

6. Seat patient before a mirror and stand behind him. Let him watch you say *O*. Now have him say *O* in unison with you. To help him say the word, place your index finger at the right of his mouth. Give his lip muscles a slight touch and move them forward in the shape of O! As he shapes the letter, he tends to say *O* in unison with you.

   Utter this *O* in a tone of great surprise. Let your facial expression demonstrate surprise. Deliberately exaggerate. In this way the patient works on a *word* that has meaning, i.e., surprise.

Problems of word-naming differ in the apraxic from those found in visual agnosia. Whether a word is concrete or abstract (as in visual agnosia) seldom troubles the apraxic whose handicap is the correct marshaling of speech muscles for words. Always select simple monosyllabic words for exercise in the early stages of therapy. Have him begin with a consonant and end with a vowel. By starting with these simpler words first, the patient can experience success in his initial attempts. This builds confidence so essential for good therapy. After patient produces *O*, teach him to say and write the word in unison and then to say and write it from dictation. Follow directions under Therapy for Visual Agnosia, Therapeutic Procedures for Word-naming, steps 1–37, pages 110–24. In beginning therapy, use this tracing-speaking-reading-writing-dictation procedure with *every* word as it is learned. Soon he will learn words without tracing them. When teaching him to write words, the following additional recommendations are helpful to overcome writing difficulties or *paragraphia:*

a. If there is loss of skill in grasping a pencil or pen, take up this problem in the earliest stages of therapy. Seat patient comfortably at a table or desk with paper placed at the correct angle for left- or right-handed writing. See Warren Gardner's *Left Handed Writing* (Interstate Press, Danville, Illinois, 1945) for specific directions. After demonstrating procedure for writing and saying *O* (see step 6, page 136), place pencil in his hand and guide that hand gently in writing and saying *O*.

b. If unable to grasp a pencil, let him grasp larger objects such as a:

1ᵃ. Bag of marbles.
2ᵃ. Soft rubber ball.
3ᵃ. Ping-pong paddle.

c. Follow this exercise by letting him:
    1ᵃ. Throw and catch a ball.
    2ᵃ. Bat a ping-pong ball.
    3ᵃ. Bat a tennis ball.
    4ᵃ. Play softball.
    5ᵃ. Play cribbage.

d. Now go on to more intricate movements like:
    1ᵃ. Grasping a comb and combing the hair.
    2ᵃ. Using a spoon to stir.
    3ᵃ. Handling a knife and fork.
    4ᵃ. Holding a large piece of chalk such as plumbers and carpenters use.

e. As discussed under Chapter VII, "Initial Therapeutic Considerations," pages 97–98, seek always to discover what the *patient* feels is his greatest problem. For instance, his greatest desire may be to comb his hair. Teach this at the very beginning of therapy. The newly acquired accomplishment will instantly augment his recovery efforts.

After learning to grasp by using larger muscles, more precise muscle movements should be attempted such as holding a piece of chalk and moving it across the blackboard. With blackboard-writing activities, follow procedure described earlier for use with a pencil. After he attains some ease in using chalk, return again to grasping a pencil and writing. If unable to use a pencil, continue using the chalk and blackboard until he displays some skill—then transfer this ability to the pencil. Follow the writing suggestions outlined for paragraphia, pages 137–39 of this section. Repeat all these exercises until he can do them with moderate skill.

These next exercises[6] were worked out by one of us during a research study of dysarthric problems of spastic and athetoid patients at the Orthopaedic Hospital, Los Angeles, in 1946. The procedures may be used *not only* for apraxics who have difficulty in using the speech muscles for certain purposes, but with patients who have difficulty in using the speech muscles specifically for speech.

7. To aid in developing awareness of soft palate action (necessary for the *k* and *g*):

   a. Suggest that patient watch the uvula rise in the back of the throat as you yawn. After a few times, have him yawn. Hold a mirror up so he may watch his uvula move as he yawns; tell him to sense the "feel" and action of the palatal muscles as they are raised and lowered.

   b. Uvula action may also be learned by asking him to blow up balloons, blow out a candle, blow up a sack.

8. Place your hand under his jaw and move it up and down. Directions to patient are: "Just let the jaw relax; get the feel and action of the jaw as it is being moved; up-down-rest, up-down-rest, up-down-rest." The "rest" phase should be of several seconds' duration. Give this exercise while he is supine. Then give it while he sits in a chair before the mirror.

   After aiding with these jaw movements, suggest that he execute them on his own volition. Again the directions should be "let the jaw relax, up-down-rest, up-down-rest."

6 Hansen, R.; Longerich, E.; and Longerich M.: "The Physical Therapy Approach to Spasticity and Athetosis," *Physiotherapy Rev.*, 27:178–80, 1947.

9. Hold a small square of paper toweling in your hand. Ask him to protrude and rest the tongue on the towel. Gently grasp tongue and move it up and down slowly. Directions are: "Let the tongue be soft as it lies in my hand; up-down, up-down, rest." In a similar manner, move tongue right and left as you say, "right-left, right-left, right-left, rest," etc. When he seems to be joining his efforts to yours in these exercises, suggest that he take hold of his tongue and execute these movements. (If his arm, hand, or fingers are paralyzed, omit this step.) Follow this procedure by suggesting that he execute the tongue movements without the help of the hand.

10. Stand at left side of patient. Place your right index finger on his upper lip and your left index finger on his lower lip. Give directions: "Let the lips be 'soft'; now open-close-rest; open-close-rest," etc. As with the jaw and tongue exercises, suggest that he now use his own index fingers to help open and close the lips. Next, suggest that he open and close the lips naturally.

11. Review exercises for *O*. (See step 6, page 138.) Similarly, *ah* as in *father* may be taught by having the patient shape his arms in the oval form of an *ah*. Say *ah!* with an amazed tone and an expression of amazement on your countenance.

12. Take the word *eye*. Ask patient to open his mouth wide. If he has difficulty, lightly touch his chin and suggest, "Just relax your chin and let's open your mouth." As you do this, say *ah* and have him try to say it. Then move jaw upward to complete the *ah* with an *i* (e.g., *ah——i*) which becomes *eye*. This should be one unified procedure, i.e., no break in utterance between *ah* and *i*. Do this several times and

then help him point his index finger at himself as he says *eye*. The word *eye* is used because it has meaning to the patient.

After he can say *eye* understandably, present the writing of the word *eye*, using speaking-writing procedures described above. (Also see steps 1–5, Therapy for Visual Agnosia, Therapeutic Procedures for Word-naming, pages 110–12.) Use this speaking-writing procedure with each word after he has learned to use the speech muscles to produce it.

13. Again, using a lighted candle, let him attempt to blow it out as he says "boo!" Stand at left side of patient. Place your right index finger at center of his upper lip and your left index finger at center of his lower lip. Help him bring lips in contact while saying *boo!* with forceful meaning. Show him how to blow out a candle by saying "boo!" The first successful try gives most patients real satisfaction.

"Boo!" may also be taught by having him blow a feather or a small piece of paper across a glass-top table or other smooth surface.

14. Now repeat step 12 but suggest that he "sigh" as he begins the word *eye*. When he sighs as he utters *eye*, he gets the word *high*. Repeat this several times.

15. Suggest that he "whisper" *boo!* He finds he actually says *pu*. Sometimes it helps to suggest, "You smell a skunk as you say *pu*."

16. Place your right index finger on his lower lip. Tell him you will help close his lips for humming *m*; then you will aid him to relax and open his lips for *ah*. Pronounce the word *ma* in one unified utterance as you perform these lip movements. In these exercises be *sure* the movements of the lip, jaw, and/or

tongue are continuous. Avoid all interruptions of syllables or sounds within any word (e.g., pronounce *ma* in continuous sounds—not *m-a*).

17. Teach *pa* in a similar way. Give added suggestions to build up pressure at the mouth as his lips are closed.

18. Teach *pie* by telling him to open his mouth slightly wide for *p-ah-*, then close lips (i.e., smile) a little for the *e*. The result will be *p-ah-ee* or *pie*.

19. Teach *buy* in this way. Have him place one hand on his vocal cords and vibrate them (step 3, page 136) as he brings the lips together.

20. To show him how to say *my*, first review the word *ma*. Tell him to open his mouth slightly wider for *m-ah-*, then close the lips a little and smile for the *ee*. Result: *m-ah-ee* or *my*.

21. Teach *me* by having him move immediately from the humming-lip position to the slight smile for *e*.

22. Give similar directions for *pea*, adding the suggestion of building pressure at the lips.

23. Teach *bee* as you taught *pea*. Added instructions are for him to vibrate the vocal bands as he brings his lips together. If he has difficulty, follow suggestions in step 3 above.

24. Suggest he hum like a motor and "m-m-o-o- (w)" his lawn. Usually this will bring forth *mow*. If he has difficulty, aid him with *m* similarly as for *b*, then bring his lips forward for *o* (see step 6, page 136). It is important that these movements be unified into one procedure. Never break a word up into syllables when the patient is trying to say it.

25. Teach *bow* similar to *mow*. Give the added suggestion of building up pressure at the lips while they are closed, then follow with the *O* as described in step 6.

26. *Whoa!* may be taught by having patient first review *O* as in step 6. Stand behind him and put your right index finger at the right corner of his mouth with your left index finger at the left corner. As he says *O*, move the corners slightly forward. The result will be *whoa*.

27. Review *O* in step 6. Suggest that he bite lower lip and say *foe!* If he has difficulty, place your index finger at the center of his lower lip just as he "whispers" *f-f-oe*. If he needs help on *O*, follow suggestions in step 6. Be sure the *f-o* is uttered in one unified procedure—*not* as two separate sounds.

28. Review *eye* in step 12. Direct him to bite lower lip as he starts to say *eye* and he will get *vie*. If he has difficulty, give him the stimulus at the lower lip for *v* (see step 27 for learning the *f* sound) and aid him in lowering the jaw for *eye* (see step 12 for *eye*). This utterance must be one continuous unified procedure.

29. Ask him, "What do you say when you don't want to do something?" Frequently he can say *no* even though it may be the only word he can utter. Should he have difficulty saying *no*, review step 6, page 136. Next, press a tongue depressor lightly on his rugal ridge just behind the upper front teeth and explain that he is to place his tongue there to make a humming sound. It may be necessary to bring his lips forward as described in step 7. These movements must be unified so there is no break in the word. Pronounce it as a continuous sound, *n-n-n-o!* and say it with real meaning, *no!*

30. In teaching *dough*, first review *no*. Tell him to press his tongue hard on the roof of his mouth as he says *no* and he will get *dough*. If he still has difficulty, touch your right index finger to the center of his

upper lip just as you pronounce *dough* in unison with him.

31. Review step 30 above. Tell patient to whisper *dough* and he will get *toe*.

32. When teaching *low*, review step 29 in saying *no*. Tell patient to place his tongue in similar position for *n* in *no*. But instead of humming the sound, "smile" and let the air come out at the sides of the tongue. He should get *low*.

33. Have him cough and help him get the feel of the back of his tongue touching the upper part of the back of his throat. Now pronounce the word *go* and as you initiate *g*, place his thumb on the upper left lamina of your thyroid cartilage and his index finger at the upper right edge. As the thumb and finger touch your throat, say *go*. Do this several times and then suggest that he try it while you give him the digital stimulus at the throat. Never place your hand on his speech apparatus without prior permission. Always ask with a smile, "You'd like me to help you (with my hand), wouldn't you?" However, as soon as patient achieves some success, begin to discontinue such help. Call attention to his successful attempts by remarks like: "See how well you do it. You can do it all by yourself now. Excellent!"

34. *Coe* (kō) may be learned in a similar manner as *go*. Suggest that he "whisper" the *g* in *go*. He will discover that he is actually saying *coe*.

35. If the patient can hum "Row, row, row your boat," have him do so. If he can sing, let him sing it. Usually an apraxic needs help with the *r* in *row*. Direct him to "shape" his lips so they look much like a square. Place your right thumb at right corner of his

mouth and your right index finger at left corner of his mouth. As you touch the corners and move the lips slightly forward, utter the word *row*. Have him practice saying the word in unison with you.

36. Review *eye*, step 12, page 140. Suggest that he raise the tip of the tongue slightly and place it just behind the center portion of the upper front teeth, then groove the tongue and let the air escape over the sharp edges of the teeth as he says *s-s-s-sigh*.

37. Follow suggestions for *s*, step 36, then round the lips for *u*. The result should be *Sue*.

38. Follow suggestions in steps 36 and 37 above. In addition, vibrate the *s* in order to get *z-z-z-oo* (zoo).

39. Review *Sue* in step 37. Tell him to round his lips as in *Sue* but widen his tongue somewhat more than for *S* in *Sue*. The result should be *shoe*. Similarly, he may learn *show* by rounding lips with a larger mouth opening. See suggestions for *O*, step 6, pages 136–39.

40. To present *thigh*, first review step 12, pages 140–41. Have him put his tongue between his teeth and say *eye*. The result should be *thigh*. Patient at first should make a definite movement of placing his tongue between the teeth for *th*. After he attains skill in producing the *th*, he will find that it is necessary only to place the tip of tongue slightly at the edge of his teeth.

Let it be noted that the order in which sounds are learned is most important. The easiest consonant sounds—*p*, *b*, *m*—must be taught first because these aid the patient to learn the group next in degree of difficulty; *f* and *v*; *n*, *t*, *d*, and *l*; then *g*, *k*, and so on, as suggested above.

41. Other suggested words are:

pie	pay	pea	poe	tie	day
buy	bay	bee	bow	dye	neigh
my	may	me	mow	thigh	

tea	two	guy	go	Kay	key	Fay	for	rye
view	say	sea	sigh	sew	Sue	she	show	Ray

Note that all these words are monosyllables; each starts with a consonant and ends with a vowel.

42. Next take monosyllabic words whose utterance begins with a vowel and ends with a consonant. Suggestions are:

aim	air	ear
Abe	ace	Ike
ape	eat	it
ale	eel	oat
	inn	egg

43. These words may be followed by words initiated with the aspirate *h*:

he	hall	hup	hair
hay	heat	hope	hat
hoe	hut	hip	hub
ham	huck	hear	hull
	hum	hit	

44. Next, take words beginning and ending with the same bilabial lip sounds:

Mom	peep	Mayme	pope	poop
Pop	Bob	pup	pep	boob

Then use words beginning with different bilabial sounds:

map	mop	beam
mob	bomb	

45. Next in order of difficulty of utterance are words beginning with a bilabial sound (*p*, *b*, *m*) and ending with a lingua-rugal sound (*t*, *d*, *l*); for example:

bat	mat	bead	mate	Paul	ball
maid	pad	mood	meat	mail	meal

46. Follow with words beginning with *t* or *l*, ending with a bilabial *p*, *b*, or *m*; for example:

tam	tap	dip	lamb	lap
tab	tip	dam	limb	lip
top	Tom	deep	lobe	leap

47. Next in order of difficulty of utterance are words beginning with a velar sound (*k* or *g*), ending with a bilabial sound (*p*, *b*, or *m*); for example:

cab	cap	calm	keep	game	gum
cob	cape	came	cup	gap	gape

48. Take the sound group in which the word begins with a bilabial *p*, *b*, *m*, or *w* and ends with a velar *k* or *g*; for example:

bug	muck	pack	Wac	wick
mug	buck	bike	wake	wig

49. Next use words beginning and ending with a velar *g* or *k*; for example:

kick	gag
cake	keg

50. Some patients may find it much easier to work on the labiodental (*f*, *v*) sounds before the velar sounds; for example:

foam	fame	muff
fob	fume	move

51. Next, the initial *r* sounds in:

Ray	rhyme	ride	road	rag
rim	roar	ripe	rode	rug
ream	rob	rack	rude	root
reap	rip	raid	write	rear

52. Next, the *s* sound:

Sam	sum	puss	buss
same	pace	seam	muss
sass	peace	base	

and the *z* sound:

zoo	as	razz	has

53. *Sh* words may be given next:

sham	shoe	share
ship	shop	shore
sheep		sure

54. When patient has acquired the above sounds, he is usually able to adjust his muscles to such combinations as *ch*, which (when uttered) sounds like *t + sh* (*ch*) heard in *torch*. Have him say the two sounds slowly at first—*t, sh*; *t, sh*—and then say them a little faster. Gradually increase the speed until he reaches the normal rate in *t, sh*; *t, sh*; *ch*.

55. For additional suggestions regarding production of the various sounds, the reader is referred to the third edition of Jean Bordeaux's *How to Talk More Effectively* (American Technical Society, Chicago, 1952); Sarah M. Stinchfield's *Children with Delayed or Defective Speech* (Stanford University Press, Stanford, California, 1940); C. M. Wise and Lucia C. Morgan's *A Voice and Diction Drillbook for*

Students in Speech (Wm. C. Brown Co., Dubuque, Iowa, 1951).

56. Select a song (e.g., "My Bonnie Lies over the Ocean") with which patient presumably is familiar. Therapist and patient sit side by side before mirror as the therapist "takes the lead"—if necessary—in singing it. Practice until patient can sing alone. Also, have patient practice singing the song as he points to its words. Next, have him practice saying the song in rhythm, again have him point out the words. Next, point to various written words of the song and have patient try to repeat them. We have found this methodology particularly helpful in dealing with patients having an apraxia of the speech musculature.

57. Let it be re-emphasized that no procedure is the same for two patients. The above-suggested therapies must be adjusted and adapted to the *needs* of the specific patient. These suggestions on procedures are offered only because we have found they are successful, but we cannot stress too strongly the necessity of adapting them to each patient.

B. *Therapy for Paraphasia:* paragrammatism and agrammatism. Follow the procedure given under Therapy for Paraphasia, step 4, pages 126–29.

C. *Therapy for Low-level Number Apraxia:*

1. Where patient reads numbers silently but cannot write or say them, follow procedure suggested in Therapy for Recognition of Numbers, pages 125–26.

2. With apraxics, number training must never follow therapy for word-naming but should be done in *conjunction* with it. When delayed until after word-naming and writing skills have been well developed, it is difficult to motivate patient to work on such simplified material. Numbers should always be in-

cluded in word-naming–dictation–writing activities. For example, when *t* words are being presented (see page 147), *two* can be learned. While learning the word, patient can associate the number with various aspects of his body: 2 eyes, 2 arms, 2 legs, etc. This can be used in word series activities: "I have two eyes, I have two ears, I have two arms, I have two legs," etc. (See page 114.)

Other numbers may be taught in this way. As each word (e.g., *one*, *two*, etc.) is taught in reading, speaking, writing-dictation activities, patient will be making associations to the word being used.

Attach a number to each finger of patient's hand. When patient Jane learned her numbers, a picture of her two hands was drawn on the page and a number given each finger. (One number was associated to a particular finger.) In this way she learned to visualize the meaning of numbers.

3. Practice counting in series—saying aloud and writing numbers. If patient has retained the ability to count in series, this can be used in associating the value of numbers. For example, patient Jerry could not tell his age (nine years) at the beginning of therapy but soon learned to figure out his age by counting in series on his fingers. This discovery gave him real satisfaction. Similarly, objects can be enumerated by counting in series. A patient may learn to add when associating the numbers with objects as they are counted. Simple subtraction can be taught in this way.

4. Practice word and number series including:
   a. Numbers in patient's address.
   b. Numbers in patient's telephone number.

5. A patient may be able to enumerate but cannot make verbalizations, while another can verbalize

but doesn't count. As in all aspects of aphasia, adapt therapy to the individual's needs. See Fernald's *Remedial Techniques in Basic School Subjects*, Chapter XIV, for further suggestions.

6. Suggest games of rummy, canasta, samba, chess, billiards—whatever game is within the ability of the patient to manage.

D. *Therapy for Acalculia:*

1. Begin therapy in this area even before patient feels a need to use numbers. When he renews contact with the outer world, minor calculations will be essential to his everyday routine.

   With a deficiency in abstract thinking the use of numbers is difficult, but when patient begins to master abstract ideas, the problem of acalculia can be attacked and progress made.

2. If patient has difficulty in making simple practical computations, give him exercises to meet such concrete situations as:

   a. Making change.

   b. Paying carfare.

   c. Buying groceries.

   As these simple transactions are learned, keep devising more complicated ones. For additional suggestions, see Fernald's *Remedial Techniques in Basic School Subjects*, Chapter XIV.

3. Our experience shows that acalculia problems are best handled separately from the other apraxias. Therapy for apraxia of words and training in low-level number apraxia do not produce improvement in cases of acalculia. Each is a function to be developed by itself.

E. *Therapy for Ideational Apraxia:*

1. Follow suggestions under Therapy for Visual Agnosia, Therapeutic Procedures for Word-naming,

steps 1–37, pages 110–24, and Therapeutic Suggestions for Apraxia, Therapeutic Procedures for Word-naming, steps 1–57, pages 135–49.

2. Patient and therapist sit side by side before the mirror. Direct patient to look at your mouth and tongue (in the mirror) and mimic each of the following actions:

   a. Stick out your tongue.
   b. Put your tongue against your upper lip.
   c. Put your tongue on your lower lip.
   d. Purse your lips.
   e. Smack your lips.
   f. Bite your lips.
   g. Wipe your lips with your tongue.
   h. Whistle.

   Practice these exercises until patient can do them with some degree of accuracy. When he successfully mimics one action, perform two actions in series and have him mimic them; then three actions and later four actions.

   It is important that each exercise be done slowly. Each action *must* be followed by a rest period of three or four seconds. Otherwise, this exercise will be of little or no value in that the patient may become confused.

3. Seat patient in front of you and proceed with exercises described in step 2 above.

F. *Therapy for Ideokinetic Apraxia:*

1. Suggestions under Therapy for Visual Agnosia, Therapeutic Procedures for Word-naming, steps 1–6, pages 110–13, should prove helpful to such patients. Also see Therapeutic Suggestions for Apraxia, Therapeutic Procedures for Word-naming, steps 1–57, pages 135–49.

2. Perform an act, then direct patient to say and write the word designating your action, i.e.:

jump   whistle
run   walk
wink   skip

3. See additional suggestions for therapy on pages 127–29.

II. *Therapeutic Suggestions for Pure Motor Aphasia:*

A. Where apraxia accompanies pure motor aphasia, the first exercises used should be those for apraxia. See Therapeutic Suggestions for Apraxia, Therapeutic Procedures for Word-naming, steps 1–54, pages 135–48.

B. Where there is no evidence of apraxia, use exercises for word-naming. Follow Therapy for Visual Agnosia, Therapeutic Procedures for Word-naming, steps 1–37, pages 110–24, and Therapeutic Suggestions for Apraxia, Therapeutic Procedures for Word-naming, steps 1–57, pages 135–49.

C. When dysarthria accompanies the aphasic problem, avoid making any issue over articulatory difficulties. Help patient to learn how to *use* speech and language with *meaning* so he may adapt himself to the world about him.

As he makes progress in word-naming, the dysarthria problem frequently diminishes. Even so, specific exercises for it are helpful. See suggestions for training of speech muscles under Therapeutic Suggestions for Apraxia, Therapeutic Procedures for Word-naming, steps 7–55, pages 139–49.

To help with the problem of consonant lesion, substitution, or omission, follow suggestions for speaking, reading, writing activities, visual agnosia, pages 110–

24, and apraxia, pages 135–49, and suggestions for paragrammatism, pages 126–27.

D. Where there is difficulty in sound formation, see exercises 1–57 under Therapeutic Suggestions for Apraxia, Therapeutic Procedures for Word-naming, pages 135–49.

E. For reading and writing therapies see Therapeutic Suggestions for Apraxia, Therapeutic Procedures for Word-naming, pages 135–49.

F. For arithmetical difficulties see Therapy for Low-level Number Apraxia and Therapy for Acalculia, pages 149–51.

III. *Therapeutic Suggestions for Transcortical Motor Aphasia:*

A. These patients can usually name concrete objects more easily than they can produce spontaneous speech. Since their problems do not involve deficiency in abstract thinking various sensory stimuli are sufficient in the therapy program. Present a concrete object such as a *watch* to stimulate spontaneous speech. Follow suggestions for word-naming under Therapeutic Suggestions for Apraxia and Therapy for Visual Agnosia, pages 135–49 and pages 110–24.

B. Follow suggestions for agrammatism as discussed on pages 127–29.

C. If patient has difficulty in utilizing the speech musculature, follow suggestions for apraxia, pages 135–49, and for pure motor aphasia, pages 153–54.

IV. *Therapeutic Suggestions for Central Motor Aphasia:* As discussed in Chapter VI, "Speech and Language Prognosis," page 89, therapy is not indicated when the cerebral insult is severe and tissue damage large. Because of the central motor aphasic's extensive mental damage, therapy can be of little value to him.

C. Amnesic Aphasia

I. The amnesic aphasic's abstract mental functions are considerably impaired and actual presentation of an object for sensory stimulation will not in itself bring forth the desired response. Hence beneficial amnesic therapy combines reading-writing-speaking activities, using concrete objects first, then verbs, adjectives, adverbs, etc. Follow suggestions outlined on pages 110–24.

II. Teach patient how to circumvent his aphasic difficulty. Demonstrate specific procedures by which he can retrieve words, particularly concrete nouns which he has lost. See steps 15–37 in Therapy for Visual Agnosia, Therapeutic Procedures for Word-naming, pages 114–24.

III. Sometimes a patient retrieves a lost word by reference to a previously learned word. For example, patient John found that by saying the name of his sister Nettie, he could stop in the middle of the name and retrieve the *t* in the word *net*. Similarly, he learned *under* in isolation by first saying a previously learned word, *undershirt*. The preposition *on* in isolation was acquired after he had developed the series:

> "I put on my undershirt.
> I put on my shirt.
> I put on my shirt and trousers.
> I put on my hat and tie."

With was learned in this way after he had learned the series:

> "I see with my eyes.
> I hear with my ears," etc.

Later he found certain words came spontaneously and used them to recall other words by association. For instance, he brought up the name of his wife by first saying his own name. *Is* was obtained by saying, "Jane is my wife."

IV. After learning a series of sentences (see III on preceding page), the therapist should write the sentences but omit certain concrete nouns. Be sure the sentences express concrete situations. Now have patient write and say the missing concrete word.

V. Additional meaningful sentences employing words patient already has learned should be used as therapy progresses. Let patient supply the needed concrete word. See steps 22 and 23, pages 118–19.

CHAPTER IX

PSYCHOLOGICAL ASPECTS OF APHASIA THERAPY

DR. ADOLF MEYER, LATE DEAN EMERITUS OF THE HENRY PHIPPS School of Psychiatry at Johns Hopkins University, once told a group of internes that *"mental hygiene* is the scientific study and common-sensible application of *all* methods that will restore, preserve, promote, and improve mental health, especially in relation to the normal functioning of the entire personality." He further declared that "the vast majority of so-called normal people tend to have idiosyncrasies, fixed ideas, phobias, and unreasoning prejudices, any or all of which mental quirks are subject to change but, if neglected, can cause true mental illness, ending frequently in a psychotic state of mind."

Practically all psychiatric and psychologic authorities agree that what Dr. Meyer postulated is sound and acceptable. Your authors have always endeavored to follow the teachings of this grand old man of American medicine; hence we feel it is absolutely essential to get a complete background picture of an aphasic patient immediately upon his referral for therapy. What was his situation at home and in his daily work? Did the patient have any idiosyncrasies, fixed ideas, phobias, or strong prejudices? Did he get along well with himself, his family, his associates, and his environment? All of these facts may have extreme importance in the formulation of a proper therapeutic program.

157

Most literature on aphasia therapy discusses it from two viewpoints usually referred to as "nonlanguage" and "language" therapy. However, our experience shows that all so-called behavior problems arising from trauma or surgery involve the loss of ability to communicate, to use speech and language. Hence we believe therapy from the psychological aspect should be so planned as to permit the therapist to work on these two fronts simultaneously. We have repeatedly stressed the extreme importance of evaluating a patient as a whole person in relation to his background before setting up the therapeutic program, because so much of the individual's postmorbid conduct arises directly or indirectly out of his loss. Invariably, however, an aphasic's present attitudes are influenced by his premorbid personality functioning and feelings.

Usually after any cerebral accident or brain surgery the first persons encountered by the aphasic patient are members of his immediate family and the family physician or nurses. All of these, with the best of intentions, through lack of psychological skills, do more harm than good. An aphasic needs supportive therapy and his ego drives must be considered carefully in giving it. To fuss over the aphasic or continually to anticipate his every want or desire or need creates dependency, depression, or resentment. We have encountered long-hospitalized patients who appeared mentally retarded and unable to communicate in any way. By tactfully drawing out the individual, it was found that well-meaning nurses and friends had kept him from doing anything for himself and had aroused so much resentment and hostility that he withdrew into a phantasy world and refused to try to meet reality any more.

The aphasic acts as he does because contact with the world has been broken and this affects his behavior. If he is a person who heretofore was an executive used to giving orders, the present helplessness creates within him a veritable fury at times. Introverted patients of this caliber bitterly condemn themselves (as well as their environment) for their inability to communicate. On the other hand, the patient who hitherto has always been greatly dependent for guidance, orders, supervision, or motivation on those around him reveals after-effects from the trauma which can be characterized as disastrous because these patients readily drift into psychotic withdrawal attitudes and must continually be aroused to attempt realistic goal-striving.

Most aphasics react to their traumatic condition by a regressing to more infantile levels of behavior. There may be much that he can do to help himself but the therapist must activate him and arouse his interests in life. For instance, did the patient prior to insult have a hobby or a particular interest about which he was genuinely enthusiastic? Some modification or variation of that hobby or interest may open the way to far greater progress in therapy.

Frequently we have discovered that by discussing with the aphasic some old hobby or interest, there were thereby evoked memories, words, phrases, which evocations usually encouraged the patient. While aiding him to regain a happier contact with the world about him, your efforts are assisting in his speech and language recovery, which is what you are really seeking to do. The psychological goal of the therapist is to produce within the aphasic patient a strong desire to participate in life rather than to sit on the sidelines and watch it go by. His traumatic aftermath provides the very excuse that almost every brain-injured patient is only too eager to grasp and use in order to avoid making the taxing efforts so necessary in recovering the lost abilities to communicate.

Cortical injury nearly always produces apparently unconventional behavior. We say "unconventional" because to a normal person the actions and reactions of an aphasic may seem strange, but these are in great part related to his injury, either directly or indirectly. For example, suppose he is now visually disturbed? This is certain to affect mental attitudes. Perhaps he now has a distorted sense of spatial relations due not only to the visual disturbance but to a tactile loss. Or, he may have suffered auditory loss and cannot comprehend what he hears. Again he is thwarted and upset and the very lack of communication prevents his explaining why he is perturbed.

Nothing is gained by yelling, criticizing, harping, or fuming at an aphasic who is doing things in what seems to be an abnormal manner. His balanced reasoning is now off balance and his actions are usually impulsive. We have had patients who, upon becoming aware that such aberrated conduct annoyed a certain member of the family or the nurse, began indulging in it often with secret satisfaction. No matter how aberrated the patient may seem (so long as he is not entirely psychotic), he can sense what those around him feel toward him and responds to those stimuli in accordance with his individual personality pattern. The wise therapist seeks to learn why such responses are coming and to help the patient change them for more fitting patterns of behavior.

Catastrophic behavior, for example, is merely an outward expression of an inward frustration. Something has occurred to which the aphasic finds himself unable to respond as he formerly did or as he presently wishes to respond. This arouses feelings of anger or fright which he attempts to throw off in whatever ways are open to him. He may become physically and mentally retarded or emotionally depressed or his face and general physique may reveal attitudes of displeasure. If frustration comes from inability to perform, the patient must be helped to conquer it as much as possible or shown ways by which to recapture what is lost. Let him try at once some simple task which has been successfully performed. Once he accomplishes that, his annoyance begins to fade away.

Loss of abstract thinking[1] is experienced by many aphasics. The patient thinks in concrete terms as these relate solely to himself. (This is not a display of selfishness in the ordinary meaning of that word.) An aphasic simply doesn't consider anything except that on which his attention is focused at the moment because the cerebral insult has affected former abilities to evaluate situations as wholes. Loss of contact with the past and the future, which become "unreal" (losing their "cathexis," according to psychodynamic terminology), inevitably distorts his logical and emotional appreciation of reality. He lives *now* and contacts the world about him solely in concrete terms of *me*.

Brain trauma decreases or nullifies the normal memory span and the ability to concentrate. Hence we stress the fact that good therapy consists of setting up minor goals toward which the patient can continue to strive. Keep him occupied and busy and many behavior problems will disappear as he progresses. As these are solved one by one, a proper therapeutic program will also augment the patient's ability to communicate by using speech and language correctly.

Some observers stress a euphoria displayed by the brain-injured. Our experience is that euphoria is generally desirable as a defense (based on the mechanism of "denial") against the too depressing awareness of their current misfortunes. Over the years few of our patients have shown much euphoria. Far too many have been depressed, frightened, anxious, or angry because they were not able to progress more rapidly toward full recovery.

The psychological foundation for the treatment of an aphasic patient is the building up of ego strength through ego satisfactions. This has been confirmed over the years in the vast majority of our patients. Once the aphasic begins to recover a strong sense of his own integrity, unity, and dignity

---

[1] Distinction between high and low scores on the Wechsler-Bellevue test involves the ability to handle abstract ideas.

and can express his feelings and carry out some of his own desires, he increases his efforts to recapture the losses incurred in the use of speech and language and muscles. Since each type or form of aphasia reveals changes in personality manifestations, the wise therapist endeavors to evaluate his patient and give the treatment most appropriate to that individual.

For instance, an *expressive* aphasic usually is more aware of his difficulties than is the receptive aphasic, showing genuine concern about his self-development. By considering his ego needs and drives, supportive therapy will be of particular help to the expressive aphasic seeking recovery of speech and language losses. But a *receptive* aphasic lacks the insight to criticize himself judicially and seldom shows awareness to the scope of his problem. Consequently, he is more apt to be greatly disturbed by blows to his self-esteem. However, so far as he is aware, the real need for psychotherapy is not even apparent. Due to this scotomization, he suffers more often from catastrophic reactions than does the expressive aphasic. In some instances a receptive aphasic exhibits veritable blind rages against adverse environmental or social situations, a reaction rarely presented by the expressive aphasic.

Generally speaking, all aphasics lose some of their ability to exercise practical judgment. This, in turn, creates a lack of consistency in behavior and likewise a wide variety of behavior manifestations. A study of the literature reveals this extreme behavior variance and we have of course often encountered it in our daily practice. For example, we have had referrals of presumed aphasics who, upon careful examination during the initial interview, proved not to be aphasic at all. (See pages 62–63.) Frequently we have found as the sequelae of minor cerebrovascular lesions, various personality changes, seeming mental impairment, mental disturbances outside the speech and language area, and even physical disabilities, yet all of these had been subsumed under the diagnosis of aphasia.

At times some convulsive seizure[2] occurring even once causes the patient to shun all social contacts. Following such an experience, we found the patient exhibited great changes in his attitude toward himself, his family, and his environment. Some patients who were timid and shy prior to cerebral insult became belligerent and pugnacious. Again, we have seen this situation completely reversed. Sometimes an epileptoid patient may become worse, despite medication.

Occasionally an aphasic may indulge in uncontrollable spells of laughter. Such patients must be shown how to regain voluntary control of laughing. A short interval away from the group or other stimuli permits the patient to regain poise. Again self-control may be recovered by avoiding conversational situations momentarily. Only by making him aware of his own ability to do something about his difficulty can any help be given.

An understanding of one's own limitations is rarely achieved easily even by normal individuals and it is far more difficult for an aphasic to achieve such insight because his mental apparatus has been damaged and his associational connections impaired. Hence the therapist must be extremely patient and keep encouraging the aphasic to help himself.

An *expressive* aphasic seems to have greater ability to accept and to follow directions intelligently than the *receptive* aphasic. Rapport with an expressive aphasic is readily built up and his ability to understand verbal or written instructions adds to the possibility of successful therapy.

Frustrations should be dealt with directly because he can reach insight through direct perceptions when the material

[2] Walter Alvarez of the Mayo Clinic in his book, *The Neuroses* (W. B. Saunders Co., Philadelphia, 1951), mentions similar observations based on his lifelong practice.

offered by the therapist is of a nature to arouse the patient's interest. Until this is accomplished, most therapeutic efforts are of little avail. The therapist must create a keen "want-to-do-this" attitude in an aphasic. Discussions or therapeutic attempts based on attitudes like "This-is-what-you-need" or "You-have-to-do-this-because-I-say-so" are time-wasters and almost never produce helpful results.

Members of an aphasic's family sometimes demand of the therapist a specific commitment in reply to such questions as "Will he recover the full use of his speech?" etc. Definite or specific answers to such well-meant inquiries cannot be given because there are too many variables and limitations involved. Rarely does an aphasic use speech and language capacities as fully and fluently as these were used prior to the brain lesion.

Aphasics who premorbidly experienced success in their public and private activities naturally present a postmorbid picture of extreme frustration. These cases can be helped but the therapist must use endless patience and many therapeutic skills in achieving his goals. He must be alert to discover all possible means of creating a relaxed attitude of cooperation in the patient, combined with new hope of achievement. We find it wise to start such cases on the simplest and most elementary drills and switch to more advanced procedures the instant the patient is able to succeed in these.

Above all, never waste time arguing with an aphasic because argument may precipitate hysterical reactions. His recognition of the elementary nature of the material being used may annoy him and direct his anger toward the therapist. In this case, gently assist the patient to recognize his inability to cope with more complex material without openly telling him so. Avoid intensifying in the patient any asocial attitudes already developed by his loss.

Now and then hysterical attitudes may suddenly appear in an aphasic. These are overt expressions of frustrations provoked by his inability to use certain limbs, etc. Some well-known authorities insist that there is a hysterical aphasia which is the aftermath of true aphasia. That is why in our practice we always encourage the aphasic to face himself and the reality of his situation squarely and to see them as they actually are—not as he wishes them to be. When an aphasic begins to think about his former abilities, he naturally tends to feel that nothing can be done about his case. With these attitudes in evidence, set aside a few minutes every session to build up courage and self-confidence, without which the full cooperation of the patient is never obtained.

As the days go by, call to the aphasic's attention every tiniest success or advance and heartily praise each one. The most despondent patient, given sincere and enthusiastic approval, eventually thaws out and begins himself to call attention to his victories. Never stop a patient from doing this. Instead, take time to analyze orally the various means by which he achieved the victory. Call these to his attention and emphatically state that he is doing much better. These moments of appreciation also permit him to relax temporarily, which is always beneficial because most aphasics are quick to experience fatigue.[3]

A large percentage of the aphasics we have treated disclosed enormous losses in initiative, with increased irritability and a tendency to become seclusive, avoiding even members of the immediate family. All these symptoms are related to the patient's own feelings of being no longer a useful member of society and of not being truly wanted. He recalls his way of life prior to the insult and tends to disparage his current efforts. These attitudes must be corrected by proper therapy. One of the surest tests of approaching recovery is to note the patient's increasing ability to make sensible and practical adjustments to his social and vocational environments.

---

[3] Technically speaking, the cathexis of the body ego is diminished and, therefore, readily suffers exhaustion.

Even a *normal* person at times becomes frustrated by lack of control over environmental situations; an *aphasic* who has lost much of his ability to judge critically gets angry with himself and the world when he feels unable to cope with present circumstances. He naturally resents the situation, disclosing his feelings by physical or mental upsets. One of our patients (formerly an executive in a large organization) would sit in glum silence while tears rolled down his cheeks as he stared unhappily at the therapist. Over and over he would slowly shake his head in a helpless fashion. Eventually he managed to move a finger and this one tiny victory initiated a terrific burst of cooperation. He made a good recovery after some 10 months of treatment.

A brain-injured patient is nearly always desperately puzzled and confused. He can't comprehend, see, or observe fully and accurately and becomes overwhelmed by feelings of insecurity. We have had patients who (due to inability to differentiate) became more and more upset and finally entered a terrifying catastrophic state. One patient (white female, age 30) had been adept with thread and needle but the aphasic attack left her unable to manage spatial relations. When her arm and hand began to recover movement, the fingers always touched the table a few inches from the needle toward which she was reaching. Missing in this way what she desired to pick up created such despair that the woman would drop back into her chair and sob convulsively, sometimes proceeding to temper tantrums in which she protested against an environment over which she now lacked control.

The breakdown of associative functions between specific areas of the brain invariably reduces an aphasic's ability to judge or to concentrate. It increases his forgetfulness. When there is a lack of sphincter control and the patient is a modest person, the inability to manage bowel and bladder functions often produces catastrophic reactions involving manic, depressive, or catatonic patterns. The therapist must do everything possible to change these negative attitudes which delay and hinder recovery. Nearly all aphasics express worry and anxiety if there is any paralysis, because they keep wondering whether or not use of the paralyzed muscles will ever return.

In brief, the psychological goal in the therapeutic treatment of an aphasia victim should be to aid him in recovering his integrity as a well-functioning individual. If treated as an infant, the prospects for recovery are poor indeed. But when therapy improves both the speech and language loss and induces the sufferer to make genuine efforts to use all his physical capacities (regardless of how much these may have been reduced by cerebral insults), the possibilities for recovery are enhanced and progress toward that goal is speeded up immeasurably.

BIBLIOGRAPHY

(Additional Reading)

Alpers, B. J.: "Personality and Emotional Disorders Associated with Hypothalamic Lesions," *Psychosom. Med.*, 2:286–303, 1940.

Alvarez, Walter: *The Neuroses*. W. B. Saunders Co., Philadelphia, 1951.

Anderson, Jeanette: "Aphasia from the Viewpoint of a Speech Pathologist," *J. Speech Disorders*, 9:3–16, 1934.

————: *"Is* Is Not the Verb for Aphasia," *J. Speech Disorders*, 11:133–37, 1946.

Backus, Ollie L.: "Rehabilitation of Aphasic Veterans," *J. Speech Disorders*, 10:153–61, 1945.

Backus, Ollie, L.; Henry, L. D.; Clancy, J. W.; and Dunn, H. M.: *Aphasia in Adults*. University of Michigan Press, Ann Arbor, 1947.

Baldy, R.: "Les Syndromes de l'Artère Cérébrale Antérieur," *Thèse de Paris*, 1927.

Bandouin, Charles: *Studies in Psychoanalysis*. Dodd, Mead & Co., New York, 1922.

————: *Suggestion and Auto-Suggestion*. Allen & Unwin, Ltd., London, 1949.

Bastian, H. C.: *The Brain as an Organ of the Mind*. C. Kegan, Paul & Co., London, 1880.

Benda, Clemens, E.: *Developmental Disorders of Mentation and Cerebral Palsies*. Grune & Stratton, Inc., New York, 1952.

Bergson, Henri L.: *Mind Energy*. Henry Holt & Co., New York, 1920.

Bernheim, H.: "Contribution à l'Étude de la Cécité Psychique des Mots et des Choses," *Arch. Neurol.*, 36:69–77, 1914.

Berry, M. F., and Eisenson, J.: *The Defective in Speech*. Appleton-Century-Crofts, Inc., New York, 1947.

Bloomer, Harlan, and Shohara, H.: "Speech Disorders among European Personnel in World War I: Part 2," *J. Speech & Hearing Disorders*, 17:64–69, 1952.

Bordeaux, Jean: *How to Talk More Effectively*, 3rd ed. American Technical Society, Chicago, 1952.

Charcot, J. M., et Pitres: *Étude Critique et Clinique de la Doctrine des Localisations Motrices*. Félix Alcan, Paris, 1883.

Chesher, E. C.: "Some Observations concerning the Relation of Handedness to the Language Mechanism," *Bull. Neurol. Inst. New York*, 4:556–62, 1936.

Claparède, E.: "Rèv. Gén. sur l'Agnosie, Cécité Psychique," *L'Année Psychologique*, 1900.

Cleckley, H. M.: *The Mask of Sanity*. C. V. Mosby Co., St. Louis, 1950.

Courville, C. B.: *Pathology of the Central Nervous System*. Pacific Press, Mountain View, California, 1950.

Dejerine, J., and Thomas, A.: "Deux Cas d'Aphasie de Broca Suivis d'Autopsie," *Encéphale*, Vol. 12, 1911.

————: "De la Restauration du Langage dans l'Aphasie de Broca," *Nouv. iconog. de la Salpêtrière*, July–August, 1913.

Dolch, E. W. A.: *Manual for Remedial Reading*. Garrard Press, Champaign, Illinois, 1945.

Dunlap, Knight: *Habits, Their Making and Unmaking*. Liveright Publishing Corp., New York, 1949.

Eisenson, Jon: "Aphasics: Observations and Tentative Conclusions," *J. Speech Disorders*, 12:291–92, 1947.

————: *Examining for Aphasia: Manual and Test Materials*. Psychological Corp., New York, 1946.

————: "Functions of the Clinical Psychologist Working with Aphasia Patients," *Bull. Mil. Clin. Psychologists*, 1:13–18, 1946.

Fernald, Grace M.: *Remedial Techniques in Basic School Subjects*. McGraw-Hill Book Co., New York, 1943.

Foix, C.: "L'Aphasie à la Suite des Plaies de Crâne," *Rev. neurol.*, 29:827–31, 1916.

Freeman, F. N.: *Correlated Handwriting: Practice Books 1, 2, 3*. Zanerp Bloser, Columbus, Ohio, 1931.

Froeschels, E.: *Die Sprachaerztliche Therapie im Kriege*. Urban & Schwarzenberg, Berlin, 1919.

Froeschels, E., and Jellinek, A.: *Practice of Voice and Speech Therapy*. Expression Co., Boston, 1941.

Froeschels, E., et al.: *Psychological Elements in Speech.* Expression Co., Boston, 1932.

Gardner, Warren: *Left-Handed Writing.* Interstate Press, Danville, Illinois, 1945.

Gates, William S.: *On Their Own in Reading.* Scott, Foresman & Co., Chicago, 1948.

Goldstein, Kurt: "Mental Changes due to Frontal Lobe Damage," *J. Psychol.,* 17:185–97, 1944.

Griswold, L.: *Handicraft.* Outwest Printing, Colorado Springs, Colorado, 1945.

Gutzmann, H.: "Stimm—und Sprachstoerungen im Kriege und ihre Behandlung," *Berl. klin. Wchnschr.* 53:154–58, 1916.

Halstead, W. C.: "Preliminary Analysis of Grouping Behavior in Patients with Cerebral Injury," *J. Psychol.,* 20:6–15, 1940.

————: "Specialization of Behavioral Functions and the Frontal Lobes," in Association for Research in Nervous and Mental Disease: *The Frontal Lobes.* Williams & Wilkins Co., Baltimore, 1948, vol. xxvii, chap. II, pp. 59–65.

Halstead, W. C., and Wepman, J. M.: "The Halstead-Wepman Aphasia Screening Test," *J. Speech & Hearing Disorders,* 14:9–15, 1949.

————: *Manual for the Halstead-Wepman Aphasia Screening Test.* Depts. of Med., Surg. & Psychol., University of Chicago, Chicago, 1949.

Harrower-Erickson, M. R.: "Personality Changes Accompanying Cerebral Lesions," *Arch Neurol. & Psychiat.,* 43:859–90, 1940.

Head, Henry: *Aphasia and Kindred Disorders of Speech* (2 vols.). The Macmillan Co., New York, 1926.

————: "Speech and Cerebral Localization," *Brain,* 46:355–528, 1923.

Hebb, D. O.: "Man's Frontal Lobes," *Arch. Neurol. & Psychiat.,* 54:10–24, 1945.

Henschen, S. E.: *Klinische und pathologische Beiträge zur Pathologie des Gehirns,* Vols. V, VI, VII. Nordiska Bokhandeln, Stockholm, 1920/22.

Hilgard, L. R.: *Theories of Learning.* Appleton-Century-Crofts, Inc., New York, 1948.

Ickis, M.: *Pastimes for the Patient.* A. S. Barnes & Co., New York, 1945.

Ingham, S. D.: "Apraxia," *California & West. Med.,* 45:229, 1936.

Ingham, S. D., and Nielsen, J. M.: "Interpretation Dissociated from Recognition of Visual Verbal Symbols Illustrated by Case of Complete Major (Left) Temporal Lobectomy," *Bull. Los Angeles Neurol. Soc.*, 2:1–10, 1937.

Jackson, J. Hughlings: "Affections of Speech from Disease of the Brain," *Brain*, 1:304–30, 1878–1879. Reprinted in *Brain*, 38:107–29, 1915; also in Taylor, James (ed.): *Selected Writings of John Hughlings Jackson*. Hodder & Stoughton, Ltd., London, 1932, vol. 2, pp. 155–204.

Kennedy, F., and Wolf, A.: "The Relation of Intellect to Speech Defect in Aphasia Patients," *J. Nerv. & Ment. Dis.*, 84:125–26, 1936.

Kohler, Wolfgang: *Gestalt Psychology*. Liveright Publishing Corp., New York, 1929.

Kozol, H. L.: "Pre-traumatic Personality and Psychiatric Sequelae of Head Injury," *Arch. Neurol. & Psychiat.*, 56:245–75, 1946.

Kraines, Samuel H.: *Therapy of Neuroses and Psychoses*. Lea & Febiger, Philadelphia, 1941.

Kupper, H. I.: "Psychic Concomitants in Wartime Injuries," *Psychosom. Med.*, 7:15–21, 1945.

Kussmaul, A.: *Die Störungen der Sprache. Versuch einer Pathologie der Sprache. Dritte Auflage*. F. C. W. Vogel, Leipzig, 1885.

Lashley, K. S.: "Factors Limiting Recovery after Central Nervous System Lesions," *J. Nerv. & Ment. Dis.*, 88:735–55, 1936.

———: "Functional Determinants of Cerebral Localization," *Arch. Neurol. & Psychiat.*, 38:371–87, 1937.

LeCron, L. M., and Bordeaux, Jean: *Hypnotism Today*, 3rd ed. Grune & Stratton, Inc., New York, 1952.

Lewis, Norman: *How to Read Better and Faster*. Thomas Y. Crowell Co., New York, 1944.

Linn, L. M., and Stein, M. H.: "Sodium Amytol in Treatment of Aphasia," *Bull. U.S. Army M. Dept.*, 5:705–8, 1946.

Nielsen, J. M.: "Aphasia," section of *Oxford Loose-Leaf Medicine* (edited by H. A. Christian, et al.). Oxford University Press, New York, 1951.

———: "Possibility of Pure Motor Aphasia," *Bull. Los Angeles Neurol. Soc.*, 1:11–14, 1936.

———: "Unilateral Cerebral Dominance as Related to Mind-Blindness. The Minimal Lesion Capable of Causing Visual Agnosia for Objects," *Arch. Neurol & Psychiat.*, 38:108, 1937.

Nielsen, J. M., and Ives, E.: "The Motor Nature of Apraxia," *Bull. Los Angeles Neurol. Soc.*, 1:133–40, 1936.

Nielsen, J. M., and Olsen, C. W.: "Mind-blindness. Optical Disorientation in Space and Stimultagnosia," *Bull. Los Angeles Neurol. Soc.*, 1:73–81, 1936.

Nielsen, J. M., and Raney, R. B.: "Recovery from Aphasia Studied in Cases of Lobectomy," *Arch. Neurol. & Psychiat.*, 42:189, 1939.

Oppenheim, R.: "L'Amnésie Traumatique chez les Blessés de Guerre," *Progr. med., Paris*, 32:189–95, 199–204, 1917.

Parker, William M.: *Pathology of Speech*. Prentice-Hall, Inc., New York, 1951.

Pastorelli, France: *Strength out of Suffering*. Houghton Mifflin Co., Boston, 1936.

Pavlov, Ivan P.: *Lectures on Conditioned Reflexes* (2 vols.). International Publishers Co., Inc., New York, 1941.

Peacher, W. G.: "Speech Disorders in World War II," *J. Speech Disorders*, 10:155–58, 1945.

Pick, A.: *Beiträge zur Pathologie und pathologischen Anatomie des Centralnervensystems*. S. Karger, Berlin, 1898.

————: *Studien über motorische Apraxie*. Frank Deuticke, Leipzig, 1905.

Prescott, D. E.: *Emotions and the Educative Process*. American Council on Education, Washington, D.C., 1939.

Sheehan, Vivian M.: "Rehabilitation of Aphasics in an Army Hospital," *J. Speech Disorders*, 11:149–59, 1946.

Somberg, H. M., and Ingham, H. V.: "A Simple Aphasia Study," *New York State J. Med.*, 44:1126–27, 1944.

Stekel, Wilhelm: *Disorders of the Instincts and Emotions* (10 vols.). Liveright Publishing Corp., New York (individual volumes published at various dates).

Stengel, E. (translator): *Sigmund Freud on Aphasia*. International Universities Press, Inc., New York, 1953.

Stieri, E.: *Book of Indoor Living*. Whittlesey House, New York, 1946.

Stinchfield, S. M.: *Children with Delayed or Defective Speech*. Stanford University Press, Stanford, California, 1940.

Taylor, James (ed.): *Selected Writings of John Hughlings Jackson*. Hodder & Stoughton, Ltd., London, 1932, vol. 2, pp. 146–211.

Travis, Lee Edward: *Speech Pathology*. D. Appleton & Co., New York, 1931.

Trowbridge, C. R.: *Feeling Better?* Dodd, Mead & Co., New York, 1936.

Van Riper, Charles: *Speech Correction; Principles and Methods.* Prentice-Hall, Inc., New York, 1947.

Watkins, John G.: *Hypnotherapy of War Neuroses.* The Ronald Press Co., New York, 1949.

Webb, E. T., and Morgan, J. B.: *Strategy in Handling People,* rev. ed. Garden City Publishing Co., New York, 1948.

Weisenburg, T., and McBride, K.: *Aphasia.* The Commonwealth Fund, New York, 1935.

Wepman, J. M.: "Organization of Aphasia Therapy," *J. Speech Disorders,* 12:405-9, 1947.

West, Robert; Kennedy, Lou; and Carr, Anna: *The Rehabilitation of Speech.* Harper & Brothers, New York, 1947.

Wise, C. M., and Morgan, Lucia, C.: *A Voice and Diction Drill-book for Students in Speech.* William C. Brown Co., Dubuque, Iowa, 1951.

Wolff, Harold G.: *Headache and Other Head Pain.* Oxford University Press, New York, 1948.

Zollinger, R.: "Removal of the Left Cerebral Hemisphere," *Arch. Neurol. & Psychiat.,* 34:1055-64, 1935.

INDEX